Newhaven in old picture postcards

lifeboats – wrecks – rescues

by
Tony Payne

European Library – Zaltbommel/Netherlands

About the author:
Tony Payne was born into one of Newhavens oldest seafaring families and certainly one of the towns oldest and most respected lifeboat families, there having been over 100 years of unbroken service to that most valiant of institutions. He was one of the founder members of the Newhaven Historical Society, the Newhaven Maritime Museum and the Peacehaven Historical Society. He is a freelance broadcaster and writer as well as a lecturer on local history.

The terms and conditions under which this book is produced dictate that pictures must be of at least fifty years of age and so our story – reluctantly – ends in 1940.

GB ISBN 90 288 5208 5 / CIP

© 1991 European Library – Zaltbommel/Netherlands

INTRODUCTION

The distinction of being one of the first seaports in the Country to have a lifeboat station established for the express purpose of saving life from shipwreck carries with it a great obligation to duty and the men of Newhaven have discharged that duty with great gallantry and honour for almost two centuries.

In May 1803, Newhaven became the third seaport in the country to have a lifeboat station established, some 21 years before the founding of the RNLI itself. It was established because of the great number of wrecks that had occurred along the coast. This had always caused concern with the public, so much so that in November 1786 a scheme was put forward for cutting large gaps or passages through the cliffs between Newhaven and Saltdean as a means of succouring shipwrecked mariners. A notice calling a meeting of the 'nobility and gentry' was published in the Lewes Advertiser pointing out the large number of shipwrecks that had occurred in the past year and the loss of life as a result. The meeting was held at Lewes, Lord Sheffield presiding, a committee was set up consisting of many local people, and the result of their deliberations was that they were in favour of using machines fitted with rope ladders and left in the care of responsible farmers using the cliffs. The cutting of large gaps or passages was, they decided, to be accompanied by an extravagant cost and would not afford any material help. Thus it was that a scheme that could have had far reaching effects in the way of providing access to the beach, was abandoned.

We have learned that the measures taken to provide cliff cranes upon the cliff tops were of great benefit. These cranes were constructed with a heavy wooden carriage on four or more wheels with a long jib to hang over the cliff edge. A rope is reeved through and a large cage or basket is suspended from it, able to hold three or four men. The basket would be lowered over the cliff edge and down to the sea to give aid to the shipwrecked. The need for some means of reaching wrecked vessels was brought home in 1800 when HMS 'Brazen', sloop of war, was driven shore in a southerly gale on the Ave Rock, off Chene Gap. Her master Captain Hanson was drowned, together with 104 members of his crew with only one man living to tell the tale and he — by same perverse stroke of fate — was a non-swimmer. The 'Brazen' memorial in St. Michael's church yard serves to remind us all of that terrible event. Captain Hansons' widow came to Newhaven some 74 years after his death to 'inspect' the memorial... she was then 94 years of age.

We learn from the 'Mariners Chronicle' of 1810 that 'two cliff cranes were dragged to the top of the cliffs to be used when the tide had flowed so high as to prevent anyone from passing round the point that ran into the sea. At the appropriate time the basket was lowered over the cliff and the one living man was brought to the clifftop'.

Lessons were learned and pressure was brought upon all members of the community to make some firm and practical moves to remedy the situation. In September 1802 at the Bridge Hotel Newhaven a meeting of ship owners, sheep farmers, masters of vessels and merchants was called to take into consideration the question of providing a lifeboat for Newhaven. John Godlee, a well-known Lewes merchant, made application to Lloyds, the insurance institution, for a grant to support a lifeboat at Newhaven, and the committee agreed that the sum of £50 be set aside. The cheque was signed for the grant in May 1803 and it was in that month that the first Newhaven lifeboat arrived on station. The costs were met from the Lloyds grant and from local subscriptions mainly sponsored by Mr. William Balcombe Langridge, a notary public from Lewes. This lifeboat was one of William Greatheads 'original' pattern. The arrival of the lifeboat was reported in the Sussex Weekly Advertiser: 'Monday May 16th. 1803... The subscription boat of Mr. Greathead's invention for preserving the life of shipwrecked mariners and to be stationed at Newhaven was delivered by Capt. Higham last Saturday and then rowed up the river to our (Lewes)-bridge where she will remain for several days for the inspection of subscribers…'

In 1806 a meeting was held to discuss ways of making more use of the lifeboat by first providing a carriage and to raise money to erect a boathouse nearer the river instead of having to tow the lifeboat the mile hitherto. In 1809 we learn that Mr. Godlee wrote to Lloyds regarding certain prejudices against the Newhaven boat saying 'it had never been used' and that Brighton would be prepared to take it and maintain it.

It seems that the boat was moved to Brighton in 1807 to make way for another new award winning boat. She was designed by a man called Wilson and described as 'self balancing' (self righting?) and sponsored again by William Langridge. Langridge was a notary public from Lewes and had concern for the matter and a particular interest in lifeboats. He was the owner of a public house at Portobello, Telscombe Cliffs, called the 'Lifeboat Inn' and a form of lifecar was supposed to have been kept there to be lowered down through a shaft in the cliff to assist shipwrecked mariners. The truth of the matter remains unproven by the chronicler, who has an early map of the area shewing just such a shaft at the point in question.

Hidden away in a storeroom at RNLI headquarters there is a model of an enclosed lifecar named 'Messenger' and designed to carry three or four persons who, once on boat, could pull a cover over to prevent water getting in. Painted on the boat is the name Wm. B. Langridge, Lewes. There is every reason to believe that this is the lifecar in question. (A 'messenger' is the name given to any floating obliect secured to ship or shore by a line.)

We have a good record of the new boats' spell at Newhaven. She was called 'Adeline' and seemingly remained at Newhaven until 1824 when J.B. Stone, the Lloyds agent at Newhaven, applied for a new lifeboat and William Pellew Plenty, boatbuilder, was instructed to construct same.

The new boat was an 18ft four oar vessel (small by comparison with earlier), was ordered in 1824 and she was delivered in January 1825. She cost £90 and we have very little information regarding her stay at Newhaven. In the late 1840s she was broken up at Cowes after a spell at Brighton. Later the Fishermans, Mariners and Boatmens Society proposed presenting to Newhaven a lifeboat most aptly named 'Friend in Need'. This 29ft, 10 oared lifeboat arrived later in 1851. She remained at Newhaven for some twelve years and leaves a fairly well-documented history. Later in this volume we learn of one particular service to 'Vizcaya' and her last recorded service was to the 'Sobriety' in 1860, she later made way for another new boat. She was ('Friend in Need') by Beechings and cost £124. In 1851 we learn of a new iron lifeboat being ordered from Joseph Francis of New York, Newhaven was selected for her trials which were not successful and she was later disposed of.

In 1863 there arrived at Newhaven the 'Thomas Chapman' life boat, followed in 1867 by the second 'Thomas Chapman' lifeboat, a 33ft self righter, built by Forrest of Limehouse. In 1867 the boathouse at the harbour was renovated, the old one being 'too small' and also in an inconvenient position. This particular boat later had her name changed to 'Elizabeth Boys' by virtue of a legacy by Mr. Thomas Boys of Hove. She gave valiant service to many vessels during her period at Newhaven and was on station until 1877, when a new era started at the port when another new lifeboat arrived named 'Michael Henry'. She was the first of four such named boats all being subscribed for by the Jewish Scholars Fund and all seeing good service at the port. The first 'Michael Henry' was built by Woolfe and was a 12 oarded self righter. The second 'Michael Henry' came on station in 1881; this boat is best remembered for her service in 1887 to the 'New Brunswick', a handsome Norwegian barque which all but broke up one mile from Birling Gap. The lifeboat took off all the crew and stood by until she reached Newhaven harbour. Built at a vast cost of £430 this self righting lifeboat remained until 1897 when the third 'Michael Henry' arrived, a large self righting boat and remarkably well fitted out for the time carrying over 100 seperate items of equipment, including, of all things, a small signal cannon. She was 38ft long and built by the Thames Ironworks and easily distinguished by her high fore and aft air cases. She pulled 6 oars each side and there are many stories of her valiant rescues, particularly to the barque 'Peruvian',

which foundered on the east beach by the Esplanade Hotel. The crew were taken off by the breeches buoy and the vessel broke up. Her figurehead stands today in the entrance to one of Seafords schools.

It was in 1904 that the Folkestone lifeboat was converted to motor power and as her trials at Newhaven were successful, the old 'Michael Henry III' was also converted at the Thames Ironworks to motor power. Fitted with a 24 HP four cylinder Thornycroft engine she returned to Newhaven as 'Michael Henry IV' and performed trojan service until replaced in 1912 by one of the ports greatest lifeboats, 'Sir Fitzroy Clayton'. This boat cost £3,080 to build and was still primarily an open boat with sails and oars but as we will learn, she never once needed sails or oars to get home, the engine never once let them down.

Her first coxswain was George Capps, but in 1913 he resigned and Richard 'Dick' Payne was confirmed as coxswain. It was in 1924 on a cold November night that RMS 'Dieppe' ran aground whilst entering the harbour. Two tugs rushed to her assistance and one, the little 'Richmere' fouled her screw and foundered by the promenade steps. The lifeboat went alongside and took off the crew just as the tug sank, causing serious damage to the lifeboat. The coxswain was awarded the RNLIs bronze medal for this service. It was in December 1929 that the crew and vessel were tested to the full; wind speeds were the highest since records were kept, reaching 112 mph in gusts. The lifeboat received its second call for help that night and put to sea in unimaginable conditions. The distressed vessel 'Mogens Koch' was first reported by the Birling Gap coastguards bound for Villagarcia loaded with timber. She had experienced trouble for some time and with her engine room flooded, the bulkhead doors smashed and the engine out of order she fetched up at Cuckmere Haven and grounded stern first. The lifeboat arrived at the scene and the coxswain dropped his anchor and veered down on his cable to get under her lee bow. At the third attemp she succeeded to come alongside and take off all the crew. It was on the way back to port that disaster all but overtook them. They (the crew) were congratulating themselves and their fine vessel when, as if from nowhere, a giant sea broke into the boat all but sinking it. Everyone on board was injured, one man a broken jaw, another a broken thigh, another man washed out of the boat but by stroke of divine intervention he was pulled back, worst of all, coxswain Dick Payne was hurled against the stern and broke his pelvis. In the tradition of Sussex men he refused to relinquish the wheel and he brought his boat round to face the wind and bring her safe back to Newhaven Harbour. The injured were taken off and the boat returned to the boathouse, where the coxswain collapsed. The injuries that he received resulted in his untimely death some months later. For this epic rescue the crew were all honoured, the coxswain was awarded the silver medal of the Institution and the crew all received signed vellums. Some months later impressive scenes witnessed the funeral of Dick Payne when the lifeboat remembered its dead, a man known to his townsfolk as 'the man who never turned back'. On the death of Ricard Payne his friend and shipmate, Willie 'Rocky' Clarke was appointed coxswain and it was announced that a new lifeboat was coming to Newhaven. It was not greeted with enthusiasm from the crew, as they felt that

their old boat had never let them down, but on 7th July 1930 Prince George came to Newhaven to name the new lifeboat 'Cecil & Lilian Philpott'. She was of the very latest design and a Watson 'cabin' type. Non capsizeable she measured some 45ft in length and was fitted with two engines. In addittion to the crew she could carry 100 survivors. The service of her first coxswain Rocky Clarke was brief, he retired in 1932 having reached the age limit. As will be seen later in this volume, he had had a most adventurous career and served his boats, his crew and his masters well. Rocky Clarke was succeeded by Tom Hill as coxswain, another fine seaman and coxswain with a wealth of experience behind him. He retired in 1939 and was followed by coxswain 'Phyllis' Clarke, who remained in command until 1942 when he resigned and coxswain Len Peddlesden was appointed. 'Cecil & Lilian Philpott' had two particularly fine services, the first of these being in 1943. It was Tuesday night, 23rd November 1943, a foul night with a whole southerly gale. At 11.30. the coxswain was given orders to put to sea to assist H.M. trawler 'Avanturine' which was in difficulties about 5 miles out of Cuckmere Haven. When the lifeboat arrived on the scene the trawler was, it appeared, to be at anchor. In the brief time in which it was possible to see anything the coxswain decided that the only thing to do was to anchor and then veer down on his cable. He let the anchor go and had run out about 40 fathoms (240ft) when out of the darkness the trawler that he thought was at anchor appeared close by and coming on at full speed. The coxswain put his engines astern but it was too late. The trawler was lifting out of a trough and at the same time a heavy sea caught the lifeboat and flung her against the trawlers bow.

It cut right through the lifeboats side from the deck to the bilge keel and drove 2ft into her hull with a large hole in her deck. The coxswain went astern and the crew began to clear away the wreckage of the mast when a huge sea came at the lifeboat. The coxswain shouted to 'hold on', but one man failed to do so and 'Deafy' Clarke was washed overboard and lost. The coxswain was severely injured, but he stuck to his post and by sheer grit and determination he brought his boat back to Newhaven and the trawler to safety.

The body of Ben Clarke was found at high water mark at Cuckmere Haven two days later, and another Newhaven man had given his life for humanity. Len Peddlesden retired in 1948 and Bill Harvey was appointed coxswain. Eleven years later, almost to the day, this same lifeboat found herself involved in another epic rescue. This time it was to the Danish schooner 'Vega'. She had been abandoned earlier off Beachy Head with HMS 'Vigo' standing by... her crew rejoined her after recovering at Newhaven. 'Vega' had been to Newhaven several times previously. The dram started on the evening of 26th November when 'Vega' radioed that she was taking in water and the pumps could not handle the situation. The lifeboat was launched after several false starts, at 4.50. a.m. on Saturday, and she soon came up the vessel. Bill Harvey well knew the risks in coming alongside a listing vessel which might roll over, so a scrambling net was put over the side and the lines passed to make safe the breeches buoy apparatus. The crew were taken off and after several hours the lifeboat returned to Newhaven. The hardest part was rounding Beachy Head. As always with matters of heroism, Newhaven, and indeed every southern port, felt an upsurge of pride. For his part in this service Bill Harvey received the RNLIs Silver Medal whilst the crew received 'vellums'. It was in 1954 that a 100 year old family tradition and record was broken when second coxswain Stan Winter retired. Since 1854, in those days of wooden ship and iron men, there had been a 'Winter' on Newhaven lifeboats. After a brief spell on 'reserve' 'Cecil & Lilian Philpott' was sold out of service.

As we have already mentioned, the terms under which this book is produced dictate that pictures and details shall be fifty years of age, so the next episode is yet to be told (it will be!!). Suffice to say that in 1959 'Kathleen Mary' came into service and saw another spell of dedication and service. Not once did the boat or the crew fail to respond to the call.

Most of the photographs in this book are from the authors own collection, but a number have come from outside sources and so firstly a 'blanket' thankyou to those who have helped. In particular Peter Baily, friend and co-founder of not only the Historical Society but also the Museum; Bob Holden, Dick Sayers, Sid Cantell and Ted Davis. Personal thanks to Miss Corrine Sidman for her help with the original paperwork and typing, also to my 'Mum', Mrs. Emily Payne, daughter of coxswain 'Dick' Payne.

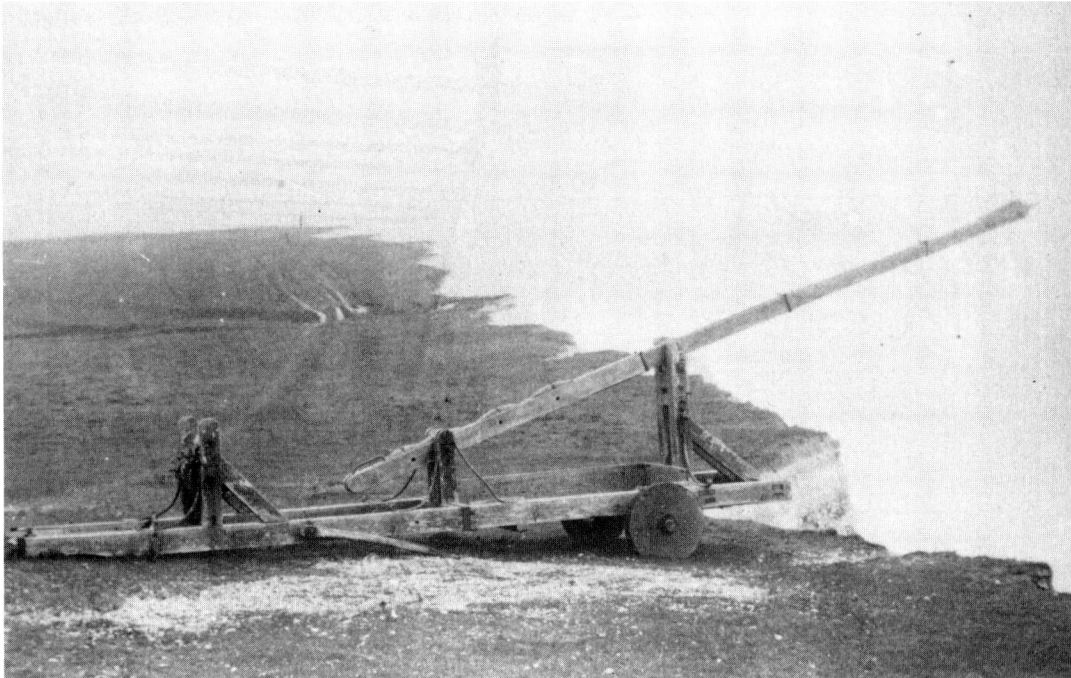

1. The loss of life from shipwreck has always caused concern and in 1786 a scheme was seriously put forward for the cutting of large gaps or passages through the cliffs between Newhaven and Saltdean. A meeting of the nobility and gentry was held and it was decided that the cutting of such passages would be accompanied by high expense and a scheme that could have had far reaching consequences, later was abandoned. The meeting decided to provide 'cliff cranes' to be stationed with responsible farmers using the clifftop to be taken to the spot nearest the casualty in order that a basket could be lowered over the cliff. This particular cliff crane remained on the clifftop at Saltdean until 1912.

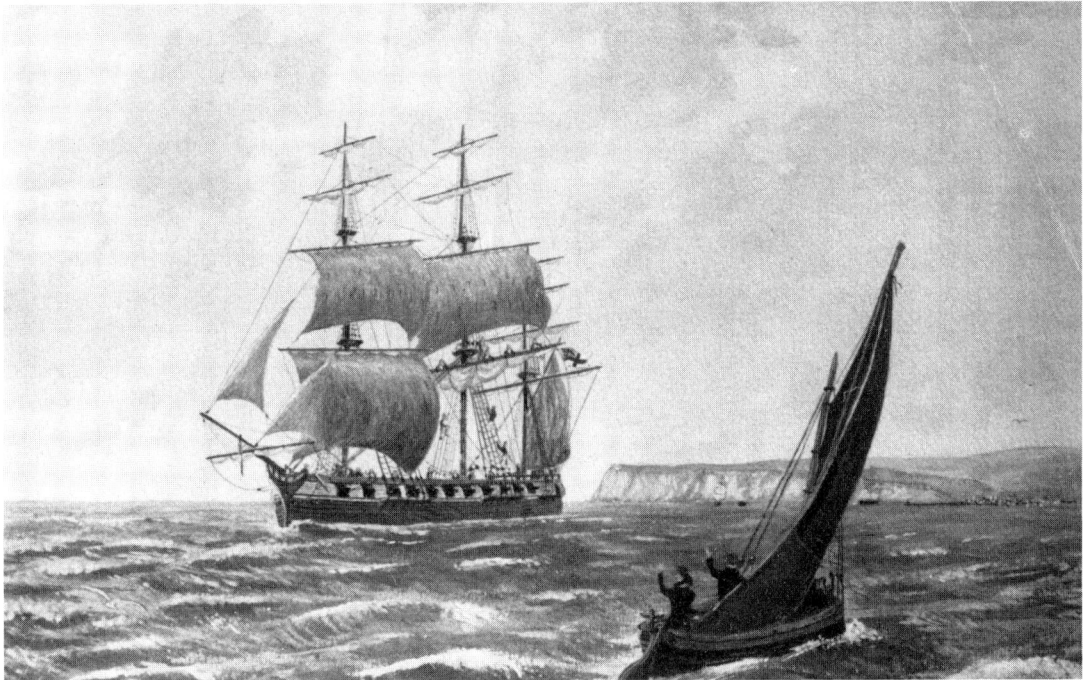

2. If any one particular incident pointed out the need for some means of succouring shipwrecked mariners it was when this fast sloop of war, HMS 'Brazen', was shipwrecked just off the cliffs at Peacehaven. Her captain, 24 year old John Hanson, and 104 members of the crew were drowned with only one man living to tell the tale and he, by some perverse stroke, was a non-swimmer. This was the first recorded use of cliff cranes.

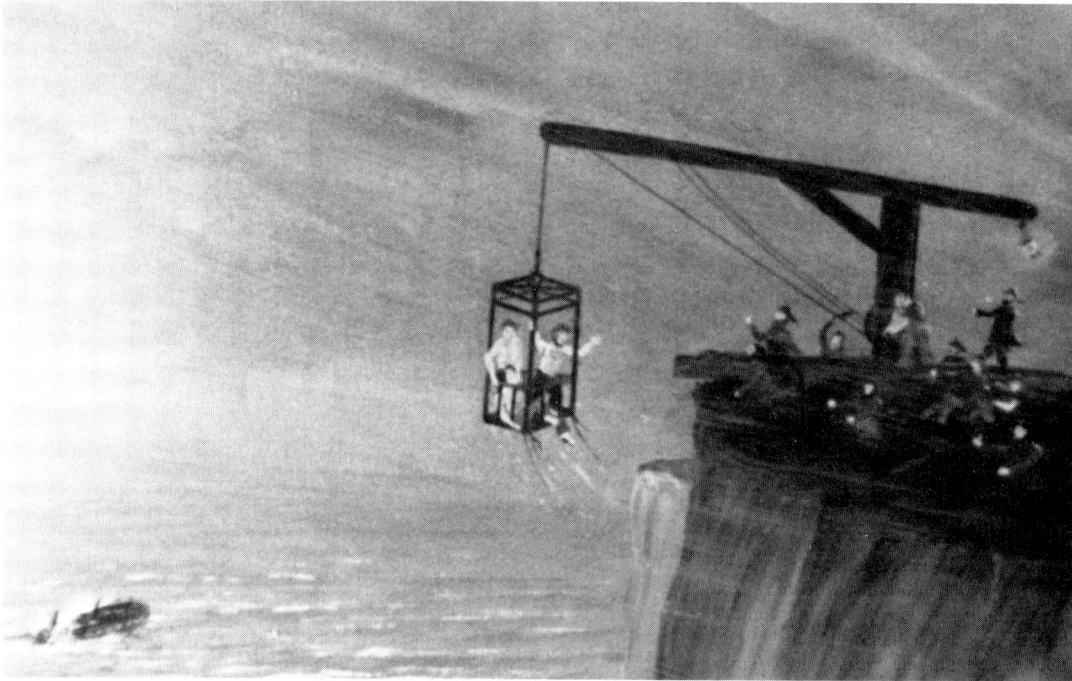

3. This likeness of a typical cliff crane by Ted Shipsey of Peacehaven illustrates only too well what it must have been like at the 'Brazen' incident when brave efforts proved fruitless.

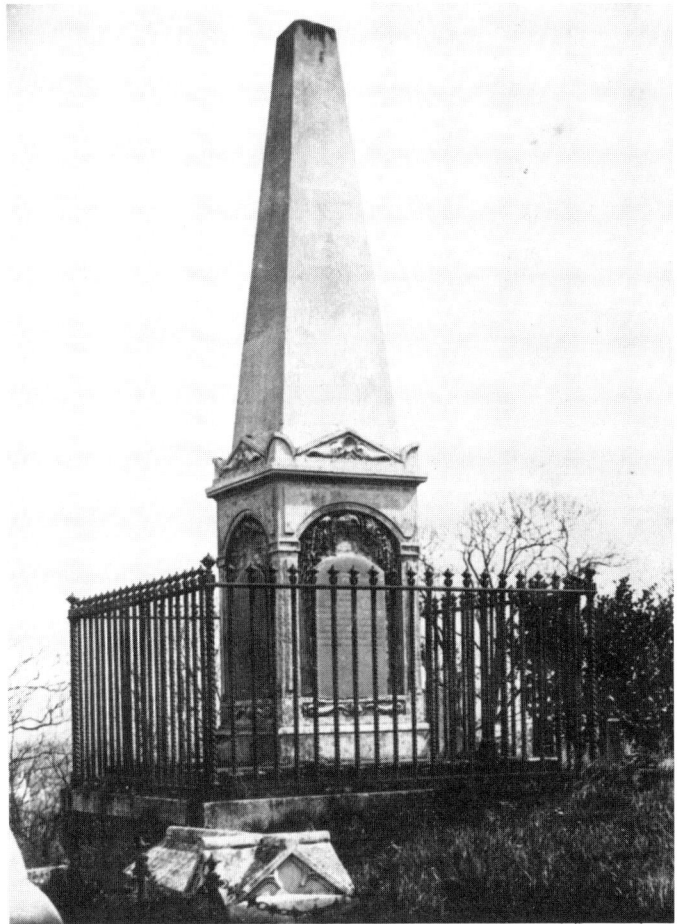

4. This is the impressive 'Brazen' memorial standing starkly in St. Michael's churchyard at Newhaven. It was erected at the direction of the Hanson family and was designed by Henry Rhodes. Mrs. Hanson called to Newhaven 74 years after it was completed to inspect same. She died aged 104. On each side of the memorial there are inscribed plates which tell of the incident together with details of the crew, their adventures etc.

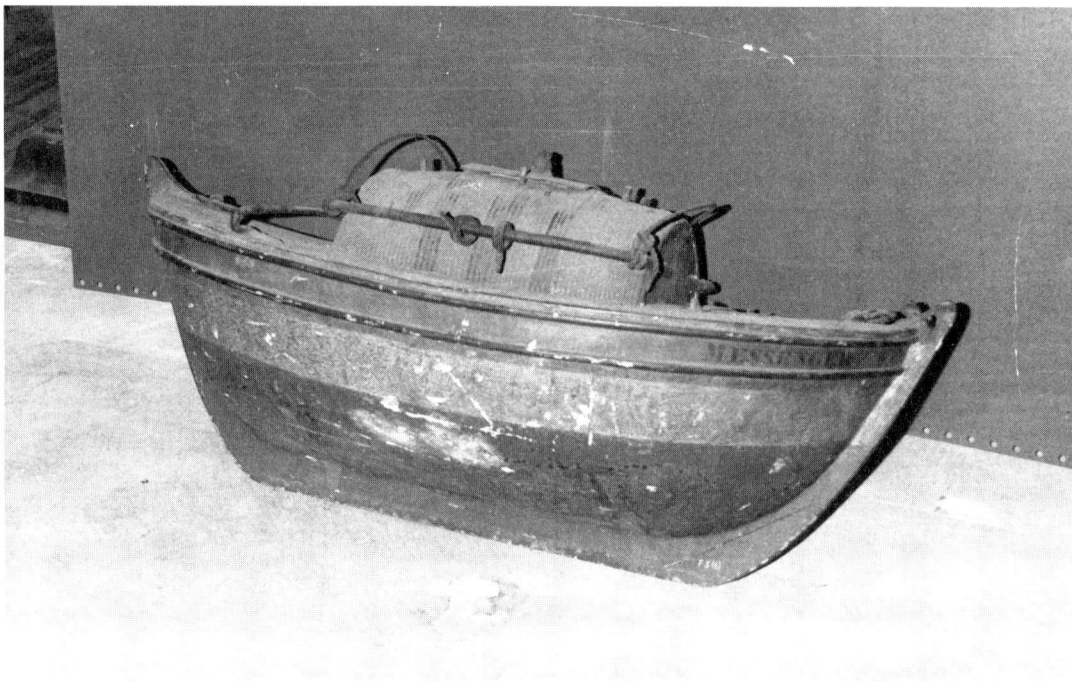

5. One of the leading figures in local lifeboat history was William Balcombe Langridge, a notary public from Lewes, very concerned about the loss of life from shipwreck. He also had a particular interest in early lifeboats and lifecars. In the 1790s he was the owner of the Lifeboat Inn at Portobello, Telscombe Cliffs, and it was said that here was kept a form of lifecar that could be lowered through a shaft in the cliff to aid survivors. The chronicler has a very early map of the area and such a shaft is shewn. Some time ago a model was found in the Institutions store of just such a model lifecar. Called the 'Messenger', painted on the cabin is 'Wm. B. Langridge' Lewes, so this would be the vessel in question. The writer was pleased to have been able to identify the model.

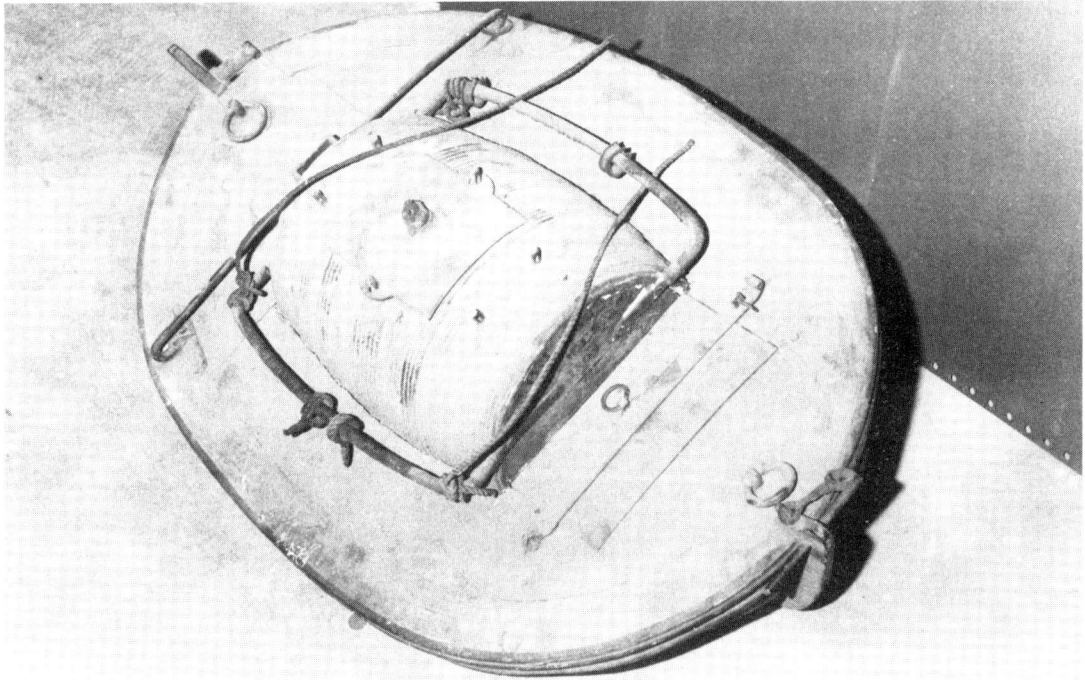

6. This further view of the lifecar shews well the balance between length and beam. There were of course very many impracticabilities to have allowed this system to have succeeded and the idea was abandoned. In September 1802 a meeting was held at the Bridge Inn, Newhaven, where Mr. John Godleee, a Lewes shipbuilder and merchant, agreed to contact Lloyds of London to apply for a grant to build a lifeboat. This was approved and the sum of £50 promised when the boat was complete and on station. The vessel was delivered in May 1803 and was one of William Greathead's 'original' pattern.

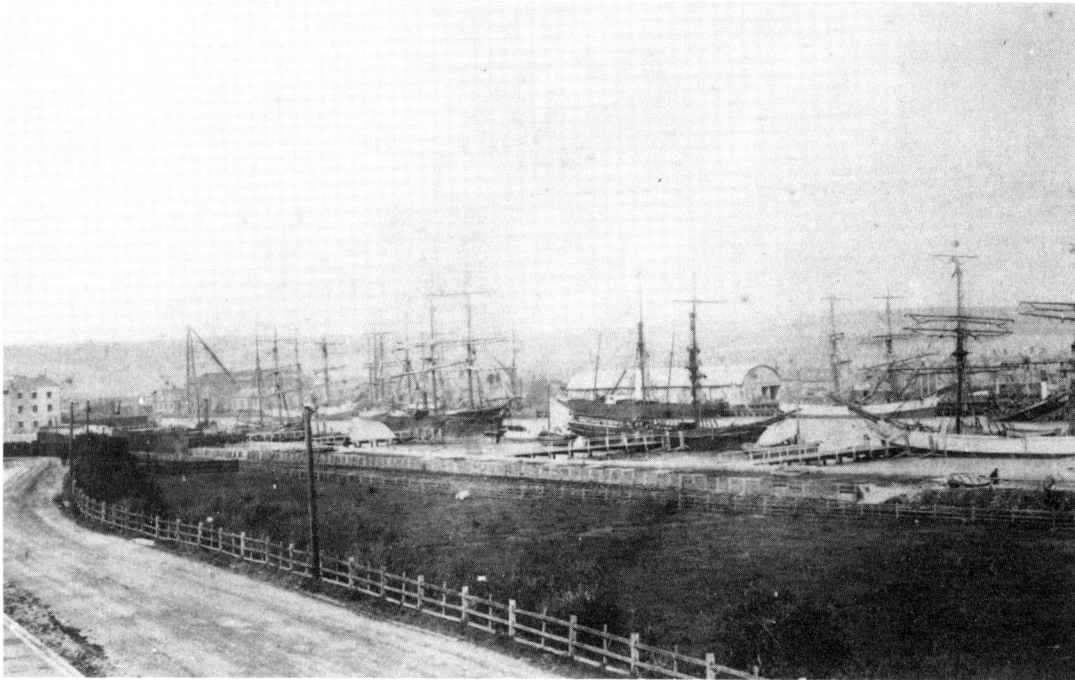

7. It was because of the rapid rise to fame and prosperity at the end of the 19th century of Newhaven as a harbour that the need for modern lifeboats was recognised and this picture of the harbour in the 1880s shews the wealth of shipping, both steam and sail. One of the earliest lifeboat stations, Newhaven has always had modern lifeboats backed up by first class crews and support.

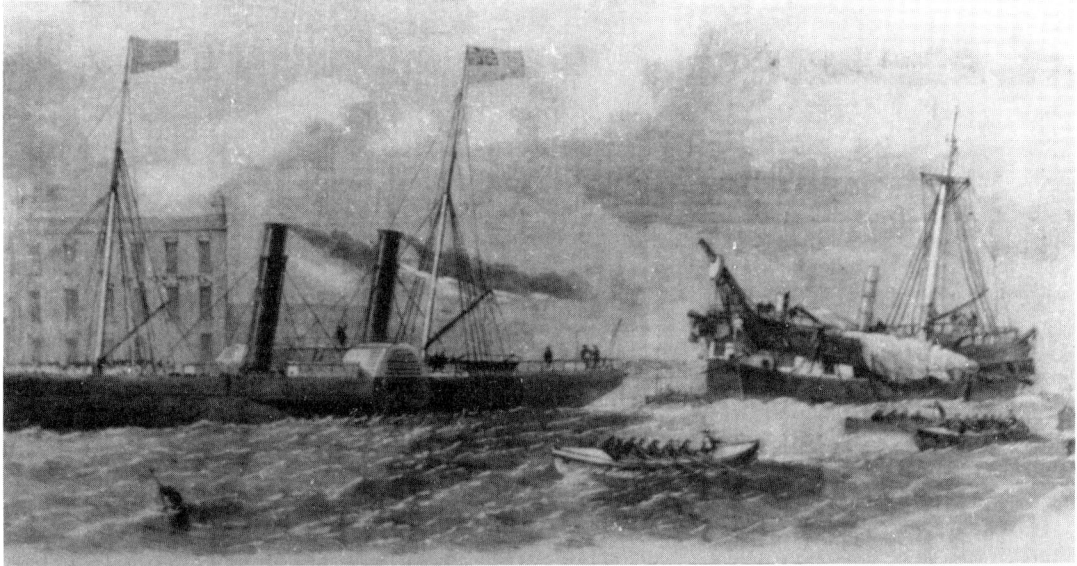

8. In the year 1851 the Fishermans, Mariners and Boatmans Society presented to Newhaven a new lifeboat, most aptly named 'Friend in Need'. She was a 29ft boat and pulled 10 oars as well as two lugsails. When the new boat was presented the Newhaven Harbour Commissioners gave to the society a new boathouse 'near the piers'. 'Friend in Need' remained at Newhaven for twelve years during which time we have records of her services. In February 1859 the lifeboat was called to assist the Newhaven steamer 'Lyons', which attended at the salvage of the Spanish barque 'Vizcaya' which was found abandoned off Rottingdean. She was in a terrible state and was towed back to Newhaven. In the Admiralty court the sum of £500 was awarded to the 'Lyons' and £100 to the Newhaven lifeboat crew.

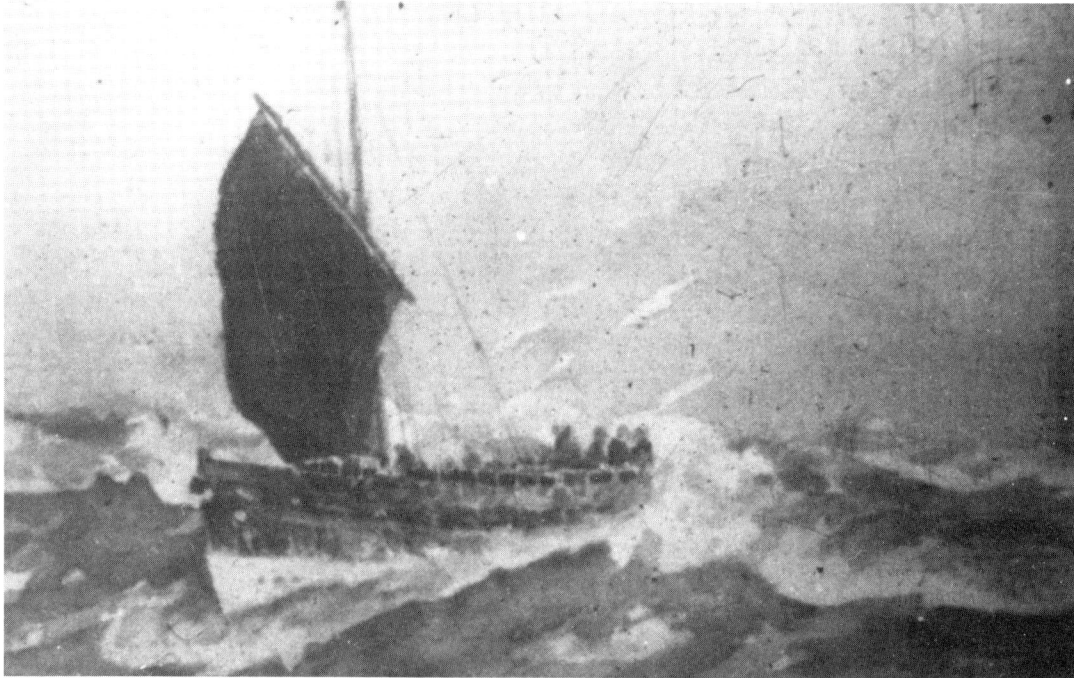

9. The year 1877 saw the start of an era in Newhaven when a new lifeboat arrived on station named 'Michael Henry I'. She was the first of four lifeboats named 'Michael Henry', all being paid for by the Jewish Scholars Fund (raised by the countless pennies that these children could afford). They all saw good service at Newhaven. The first was built by 'Woolfe' and was a 12 oared self righter. In those early days Newhaven as a harbour was considered little more than a ditch and we learn that on 5th January 1877 a barque was seen in the bay (Seaford) shewing signs of distress. The lifeboat was launched and tow lines were attached to tow her to the sea. On reaching the harbour they found 'no water' and were unable to proceed. The vessel was wrecked, but had the lifeboat been able to reach the sea, she may well have been saved.

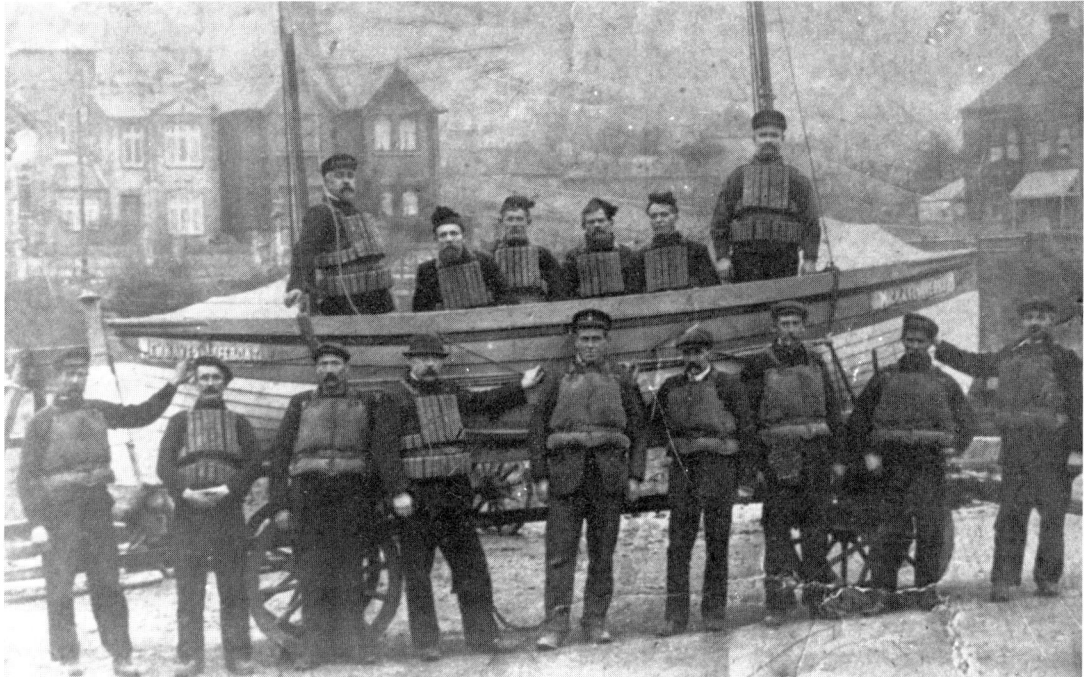

10. Almost as soon as there was a lifeboat service there was a committee set up to raise funds to support them. These 'local' committees did trojan work (and still do) raising funds to run their station, funds for the RNLI out in all weathers. Without the fundraisers there would be no Lifeboat Institution as we know it, being dependant on voluntary contributions. The crews would also join in whenever possible, particularly on fete days, holidays etc. At Newhaven the earlier crews would borrow the ships lifeboat from the old tug 'Alert' and dress her up as their own vessel and then parade through the streets to raise money.

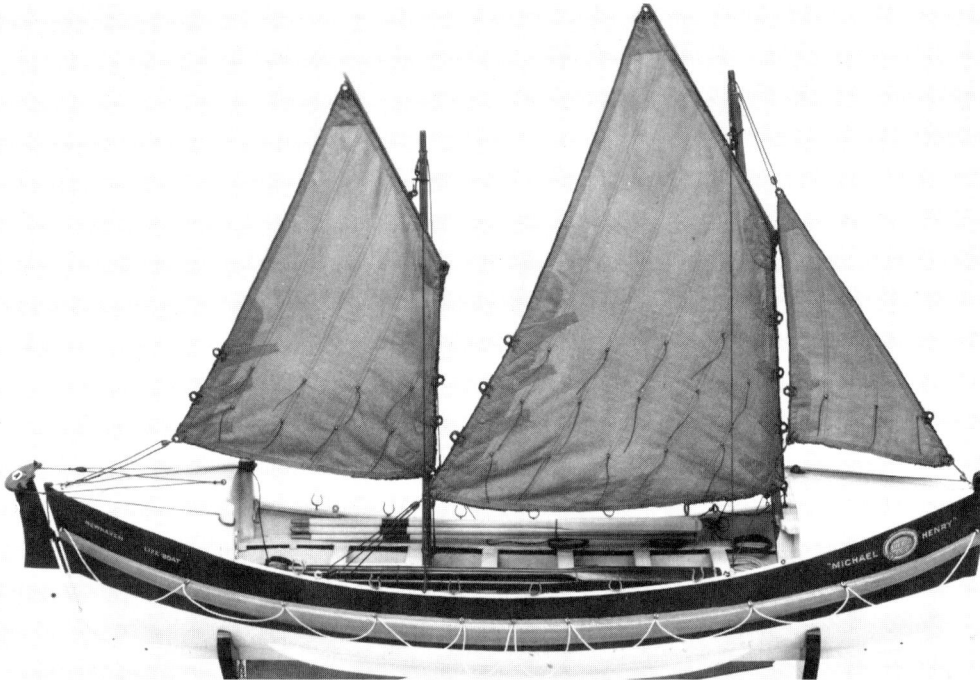

11. This very fine model, to be found in the Maritime Museum at Greenwich, is of the Newhaven lifeboat 'Michael Henry III'. She arrived on station on 15th November 1897 and she was, for her time, particularly well fitted out carrying up to 100 seperate items of equipment including, of all things, a signal cannon! Look well at the picture and in your mind look at the real thing — with her full crew of 12/14, add another 70 survivors, where on earth did they all go. Still — if you are being rescued from certain death, who minds how crowded you are. Wooden ship and iron men indeed!

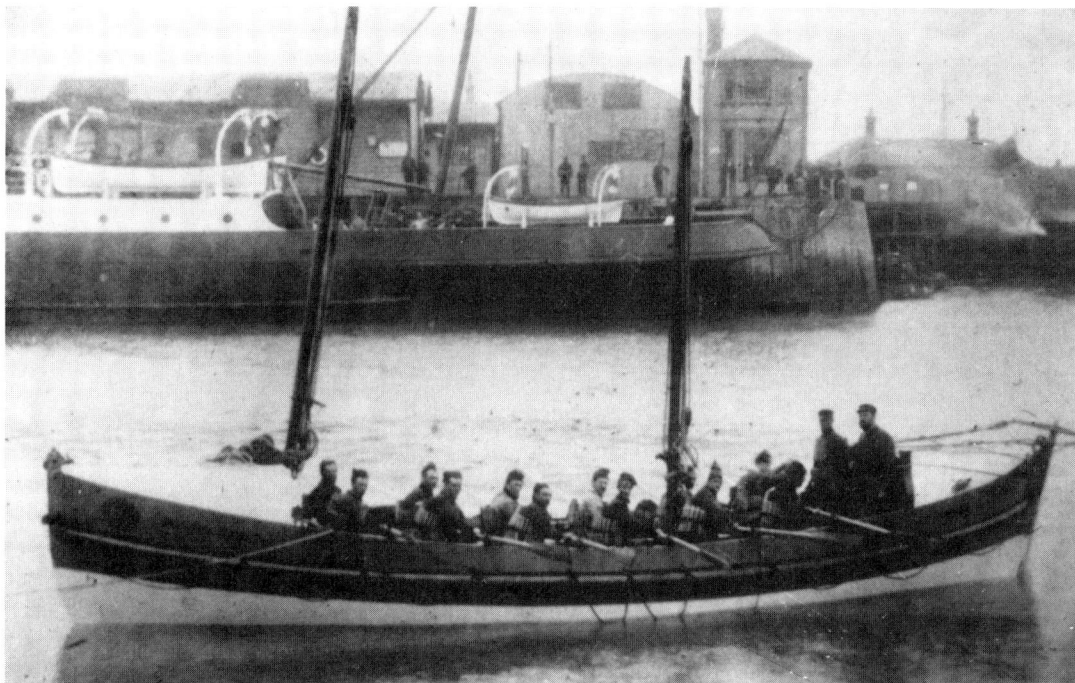

12. 'Michael Henry III' arrived on station in November 1897. She was to be the last of the 'pulling and sailing lifeboats' stationed at Newhaven. She was a 38ft self righting boat built by Thames Iron Works and easily distinguished by her high fore and aft self righting chambers. Designed for use under sail and oar she pulled six oars each side and was fitted with two large drop keels. These were the days of 'wooden ships and iron men'. Who would go to sea in such a craft in a full gale? She is best remembered for her service to the barque 'Peruvian', which ran aground opposite the old 'Esplanade' hotel at Seaford. It was after successful tests with the old Folkestone lifeboat in 1904 at Newhaven that 'Michael Henry III' was selected for further trials and in 1905 she was fitted with a 4 cylinder Thornycroft motor and gave excellent results. She returned to Newhaven in 1906 as 'Michael Henry IV'.

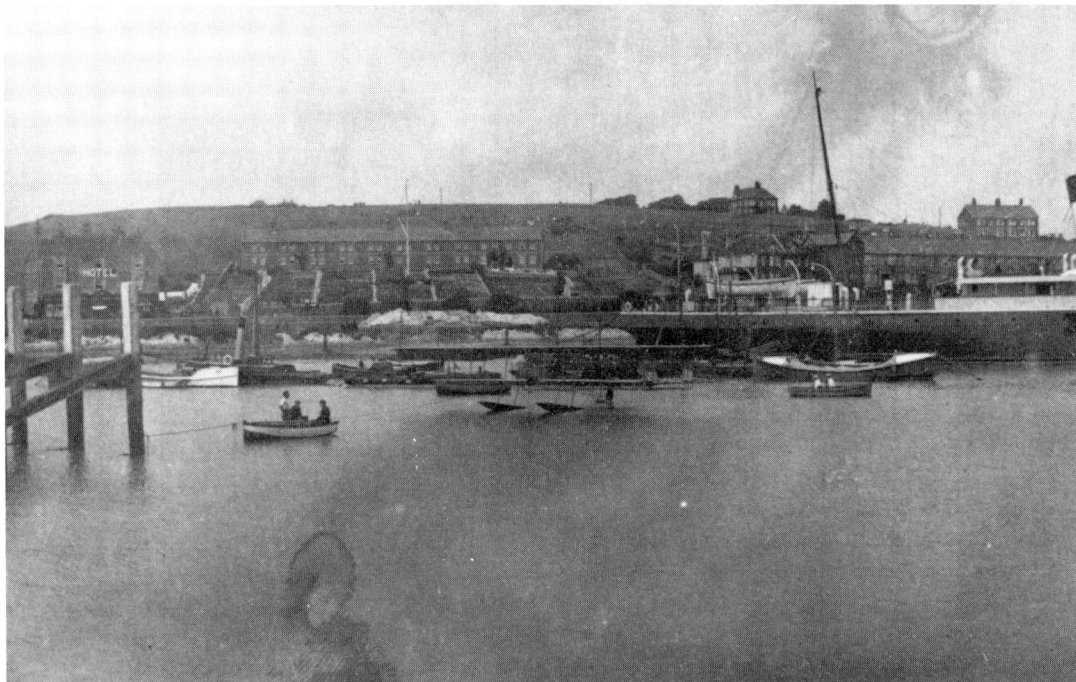

13. This unique photograph shews in the background the reserve lifeboat 'Quiver', ex-Margate No. 1 lifeboat. She saw service at Newhaven whilst 'Michael Henry III' was being converted to motor power. Seen in the foreground is Claud Graham White's seaplane in which he flew around the coast of Britain in those worrying pre-First World War days, exhorting 'Britain awake'... a warning of the rise of German power in Europe. 'Quiver' had a number of good services, including one to the 'Millgate' of Manchester, where the entire crew were taken off and another to a French fishing boat TR 47 which was stranded outside of the harbour entrance.

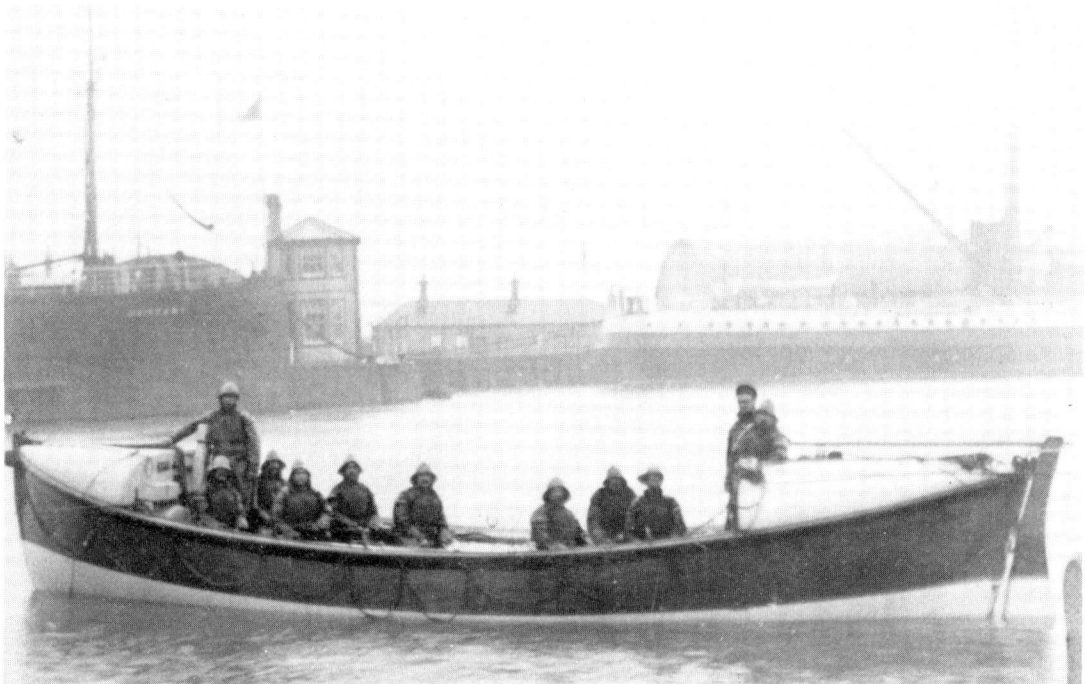

14. We have already learned that 'Michael Henry IV' was one of the very earliest motor lifeboats in the country. She remained at Newhaven until 1912 and was easily recognised by her high air cases, left over from the 'Michael Henry III' but also by the long tiller bar which replaced the earlier 'yoke' system of steering. She is best remembered for her service to the P&O Liner 'Oceana' which had been run down off Beachy Head by a sailing ship, 'Pisagua'. 'Oceana' eventually sank with many of the crew being taken off by the Newhaven/Dieppe service ferry 'Sussex', as well as the Newhaven lifeboat. 'Oceana' was carrying a large amount of bullion which was later recovered by the Maritime Salvors vessel 'Ranger'.

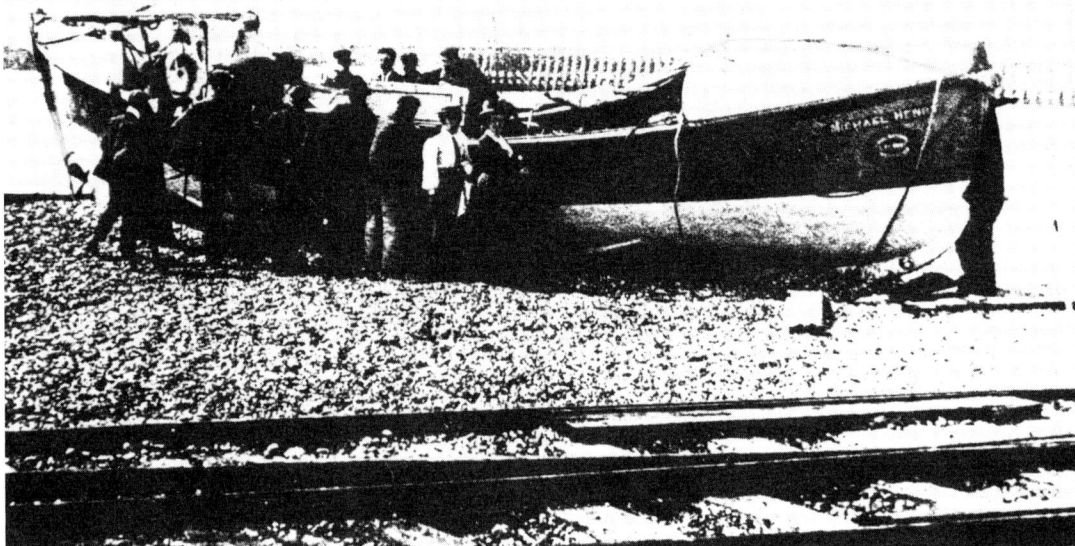

15. The steam Trawler 'Gamecock' was driven ashore on the east beach in a southerly gale on 1st September 1908. The newly converted lifeboat 'Michael Henry III' – now 'Michael Henry IV' – suffered the rare indignity of an engine failure and although rowed to the casualty, on the way back she fouled a groyne and capsized. She righted hereself and there was no loss of life. To date 'Gamecock' had had a very interesting history; in 1904 she was one of the fleet of steam drifters that was fired upon by the Russian battle fleet who mistook them for hostile ships. (Russian forces were on their way to Japanese waters at the time of the Sino Russo war.)

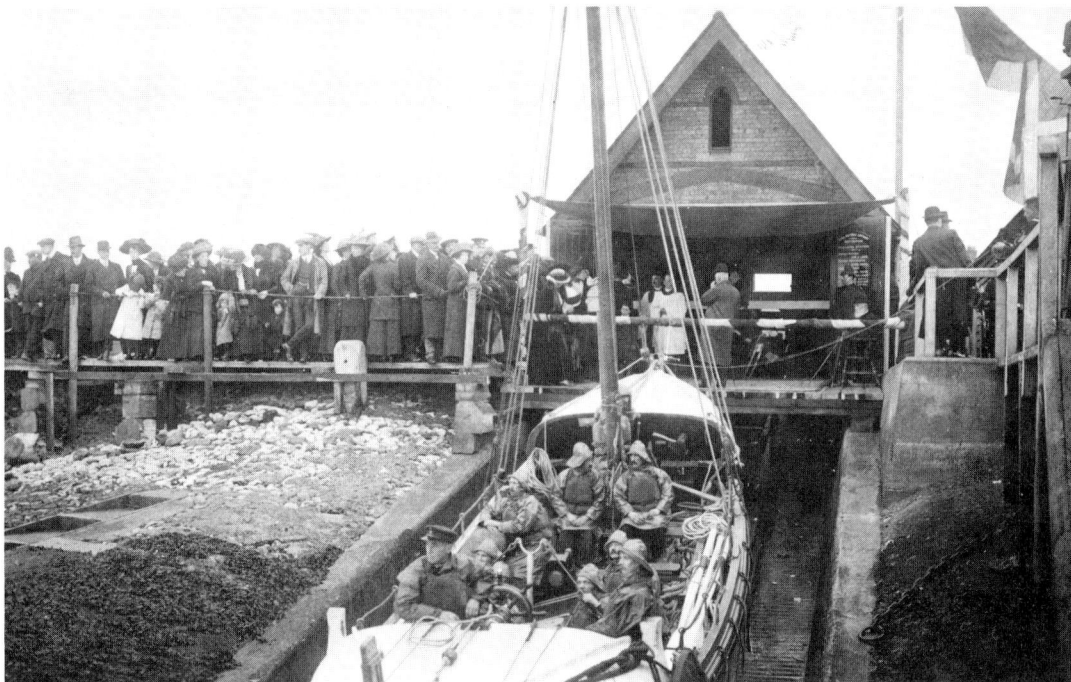

16. Depicted here is the naming ceremony of the new motor lifeboat 'Sir Fitzroy Clayton', named after a very loyal servant of the RNLI. She came into service in 1912 and her record is one that any station can be proud of. Her prodigious feats make story book reading, stamped with valour and courage. 'Sir Fitzroy Clayton' was primarily an open boat with sails and oars. The engine was a six cylinder Tylor, positioned amidships, and it was here that a very rudimentary 'shelter' was provided for the engineer. She was built at a cost of £3.081 and was the epitome of progress.

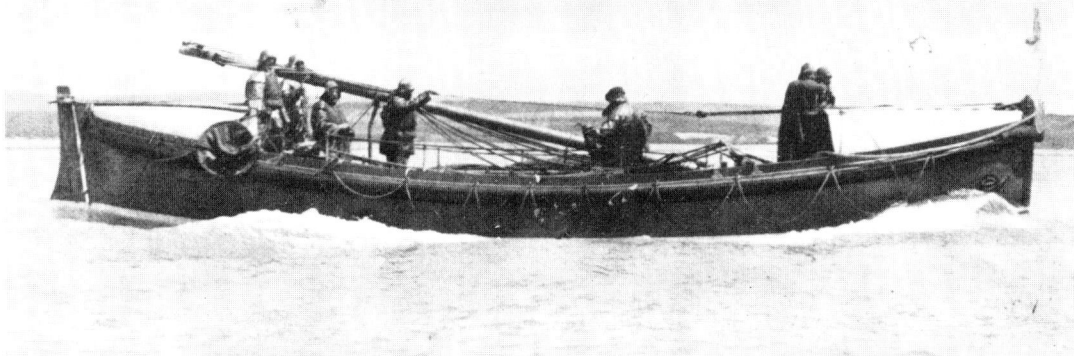

17. The lack of any form of shelter in this particular lifeboat can be clearly seen in this fine shot of 'Sir Fitzroy Clayton' on exercise. There is very little freeboard and one can imagine what it must have been like going to sea in a full gale! Built by Thames Ironworks, she had a speed of 7 knots and was very reliable, we learn. At the end of her service, when the new boat was proposed, engineer Ernie Cantell said 'the engine has never once let us down and we've never put up sail, or put out oar to get us home'... praise indeed. In service from 1912 to 1930.

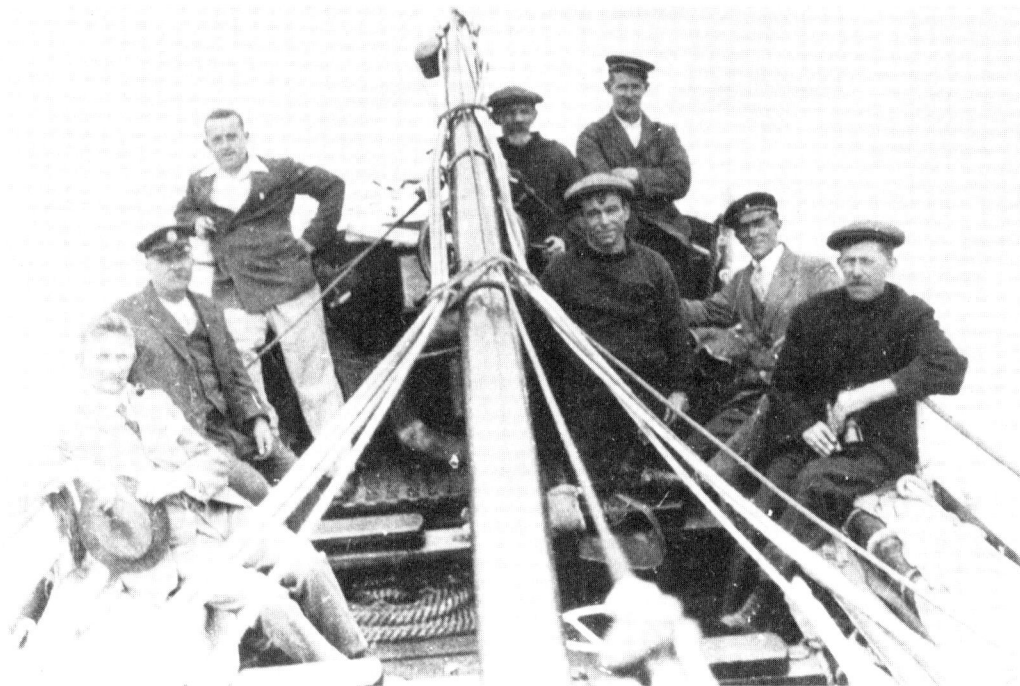

18. As we have already seen, 'Sir Fitzroy Clayton' was a small lifeboat by modern standards and her lack of room on board can be seen from this picture taken at sea. The occasion was a visit from a local yacht club and both members and crew seemed to have had an agreeable time. Looking from the camera we see in the nautical cap engineer 'Ernie' Cantell, on the right (their port) in front with the binoculars is Fred Parker, holding the mast is one of the boats long serving members 'Buff' Jones, at the wheel is the second coxswain 'Rocky' Clarke and alongside him is coxswain Dick Payne.

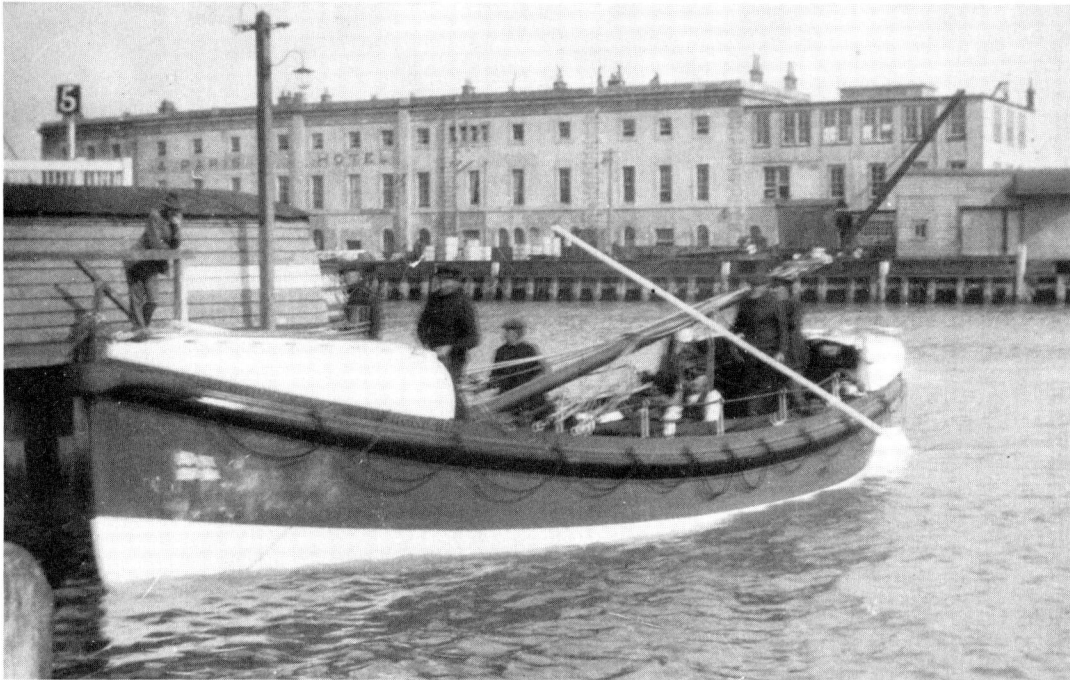

19. The well-proportioned lines of the boat can be clearly seen here and as we have already learned she was a fine sea boat. Bob Holden, for many years indeed the 'head launcher' of a number of Newhaven boats, tells us that he started his working life with engineer 'Ernie' Cantell in his boatbuilding yard at Newhaven. He and Mr. Cantell attended the boathouse every evening to 'swing' the engine and make sure that all was in order. The crew at this time was made up of a variety of people from differing trades and professions: some fishermen, some seamen, coal porters from the company's coal yard etc. The coal porters were, by virtue of the job they did, covered in coal dust and Bob Holden say they often put to sea looking like the Black and White minstrells.

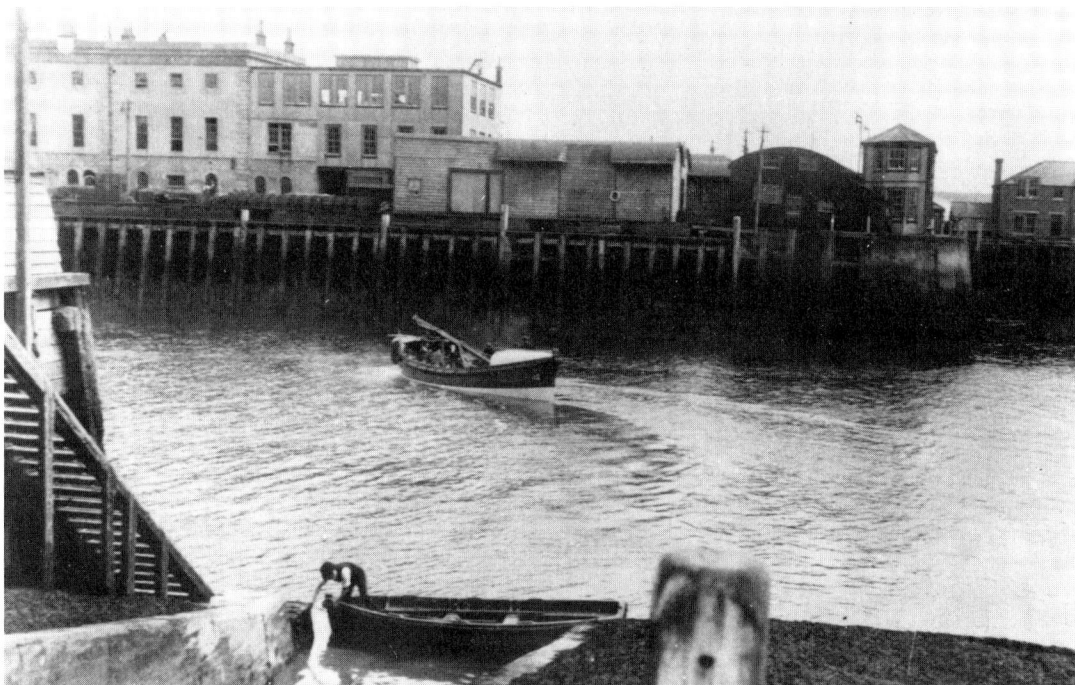

20. 'Sir Fitzroy Clayton' was always launched stern first and this in itself must have provided a lot of problems avoiding damage to her vulnerable rudder. The writer once asked the head launcher, Bob Holden, why it was that they launched stern first and his terse reply was 'because the old man says so'.

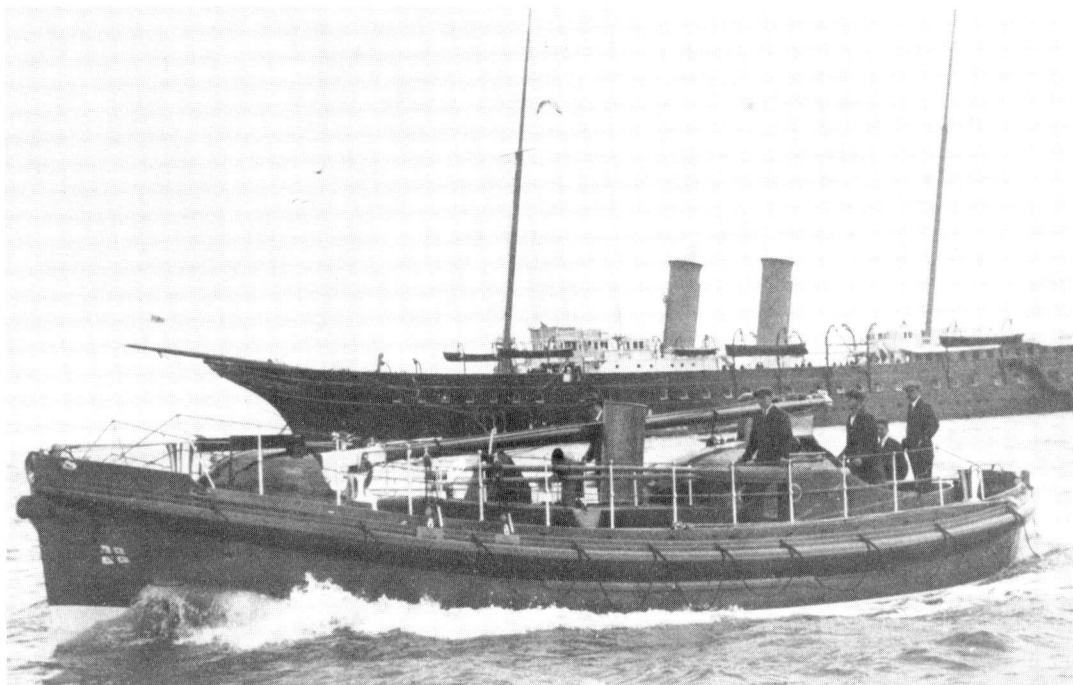

21. Prior to delivery to Newhaven, the new lifeboat 'Cecil & Lilian Philpott' completes her trials off the Isle of Wight and is seen here steaming at speed and passing the old Royal yacht 'Victoria & Albert'. The lifeboat was capable of steaming at 8½ knots. She was built with funds from a legacy of Mrs. Lilian Philpott.

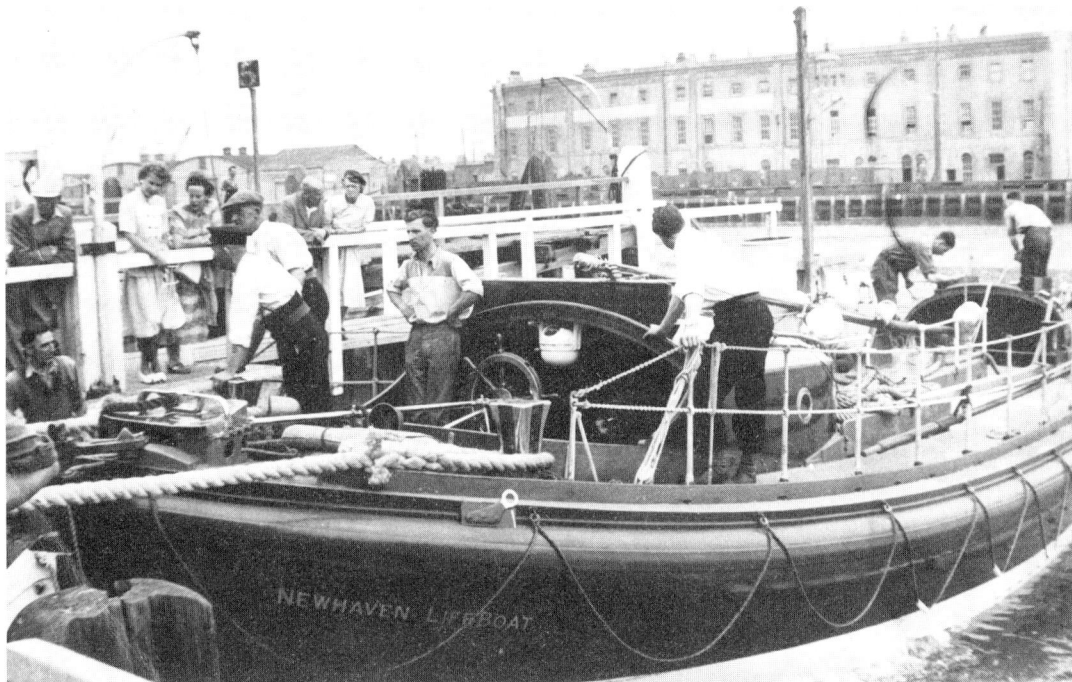

22. The new lifeboat (1930-1959) 'Cecil & Lilian Philpott' was built at Cowes by the old-established firm of Samuel White. She was (then) of the first designs known as 'Watson cabin class'. She was non capsizeable. Some 45ft in length and fitted with twin engines she had a radius of operation of some 210 miles and could remain at sea for some 15 hours without refuelling. She cost some £7,892 to build and saw good service at Newhaven before being 'sold out'.

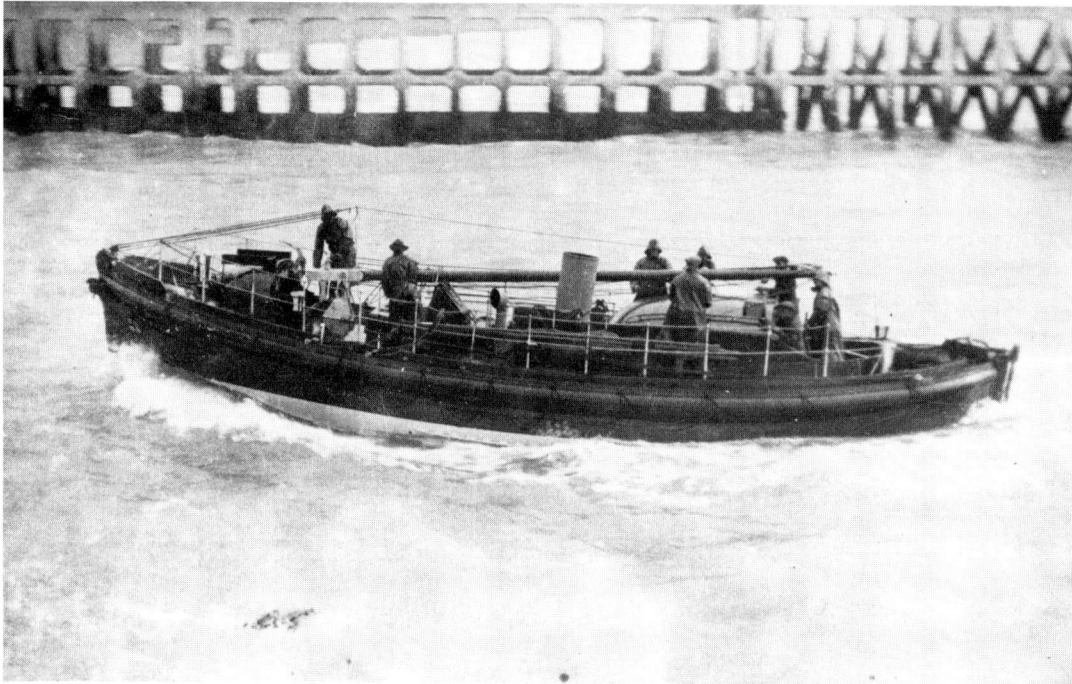

23. This is a fine shot of 'Cecil & Lilian Philpott' returning from service. She was built to incorporate all the latest technology and could carry over 100 survivors. When the RNLI announced that Newhaven was to have a new lifeboat it was not greeted with the enthusiasm one might think. The old engineer 'Ernie' Cantell, a long serving lifeboatman, said 'there is nothing wrong with our old boat, we have never once had to put out oar or put up sail to get us home'. After a few months on station he, like many others, changed his mind.

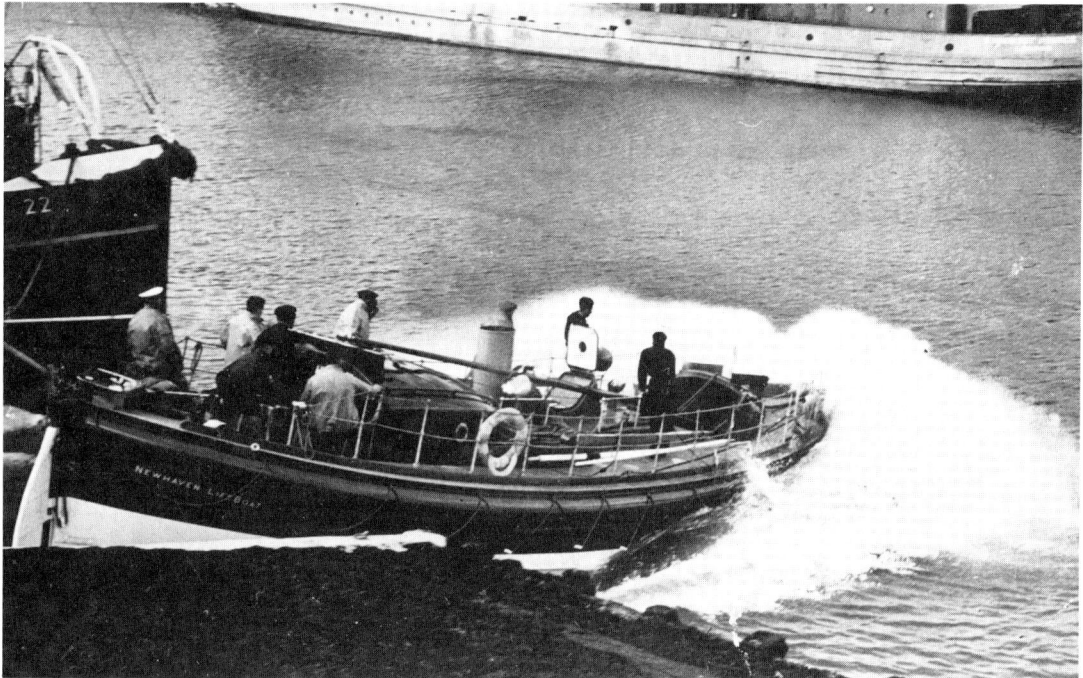

24. A good shot of a high water launch of 'Cecil & Lilian Philpott'. She was well-used during her period of service and her crew had great faith in her. The RNLI did experiment with 'steam' lifeboats for a time, but Newhaven never had one.

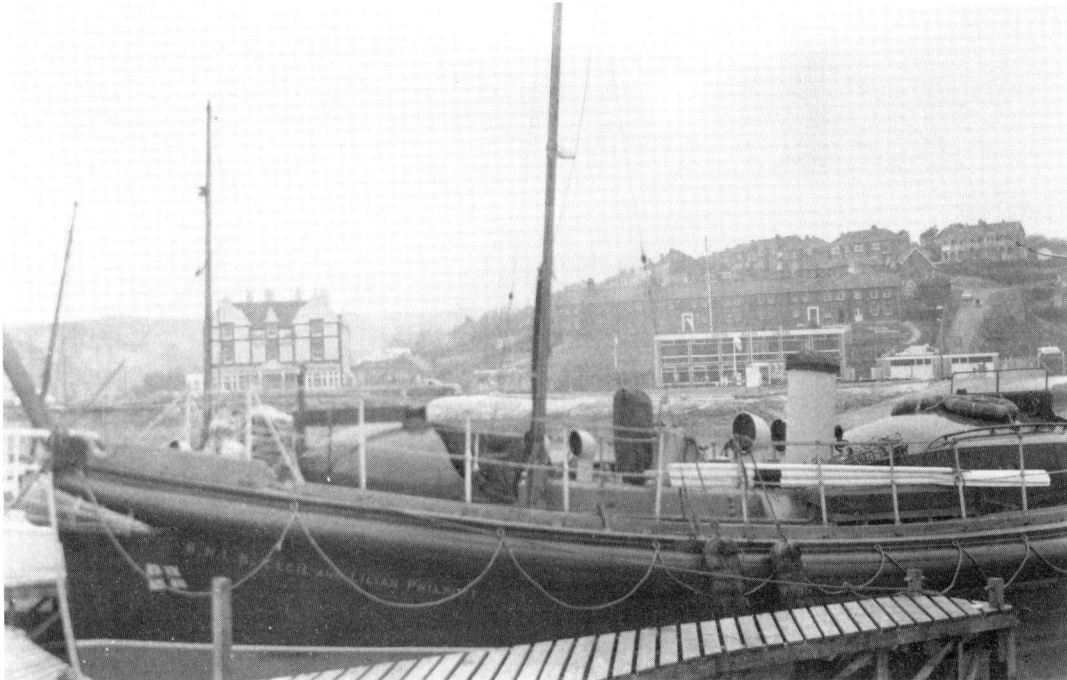

25. When Institution boats are sold 'out of service' there is always a big demand for them from the public. They were very well built, very well maintained and possessed great strength and endurance plus they were well treated. Here we see 'Cecil & Lilian Philpott' at Newhaven, in retirement just before embarking on a round the world trip.

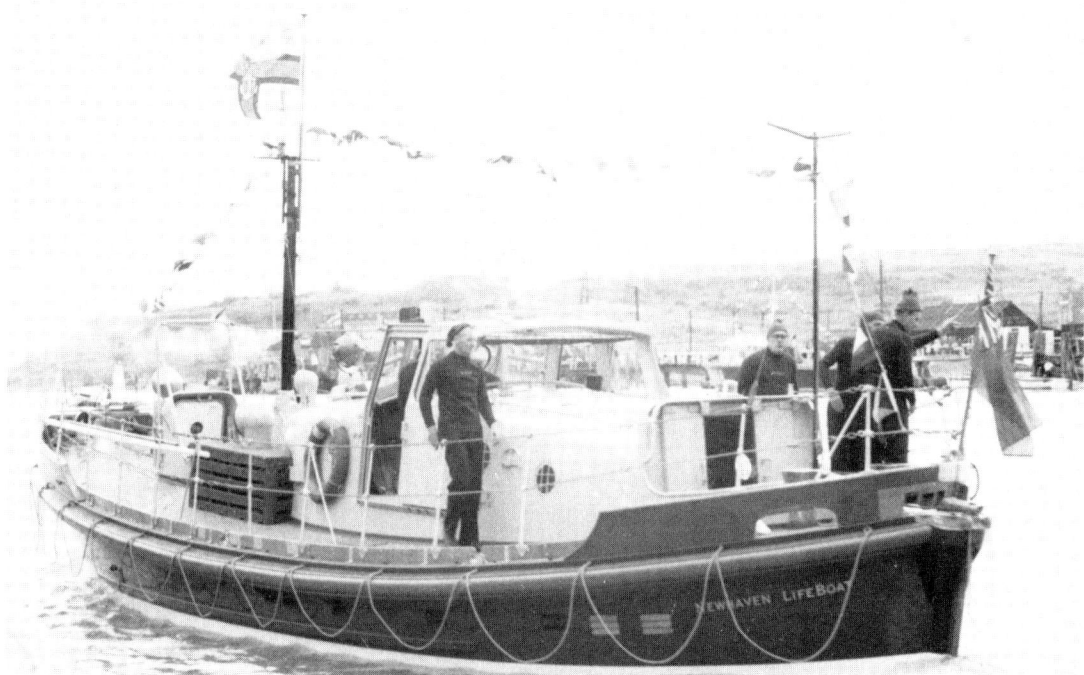

26. The publishers terms of reference dictate that pictures should be at least fifty years old but in this instance it would be very wrong of the chronicler not to include the 'Kathleen Mary' lifeboat which came into service when 'Cecil & Lilian Philpott' was sold out. She was the gift of an anonymous donor. Costing some £37,000 to build she was constructed at the William Osborne yard. She was a 47ft Watson cabin class with 2 diesel engines and had a speed of 8½ knots. She was deemed to be unsinkable but she was not self righting. Seen here at the naming ceremony she was a fine example of the builders craft.

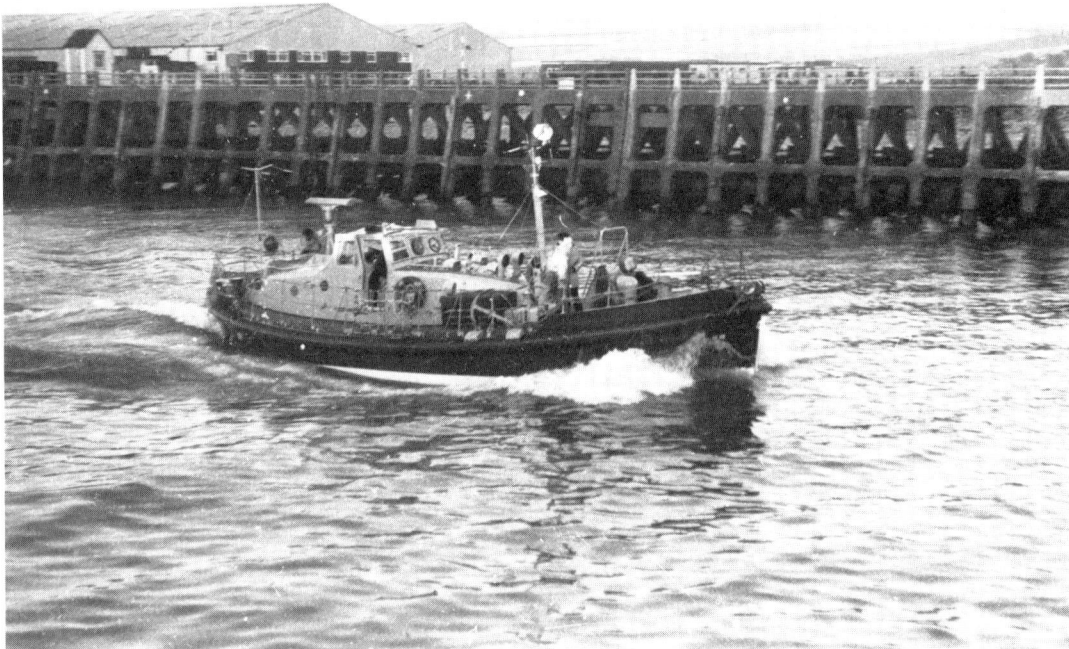

27. The fine lines of 'Kathleen Mary' are seen well here as she is launched on service. She had a radius of some 250 miles at cruising speed and 140 miles at full speed. She was divided into ten watertight compartments and had numerous air cases. Like all of her predecessors she has taken part in many fine services. For her service period at Newhaven she was under the command of coxswain Edgar Moore, a much respected lifeboatman, whose ability in handling his boat was legendary.

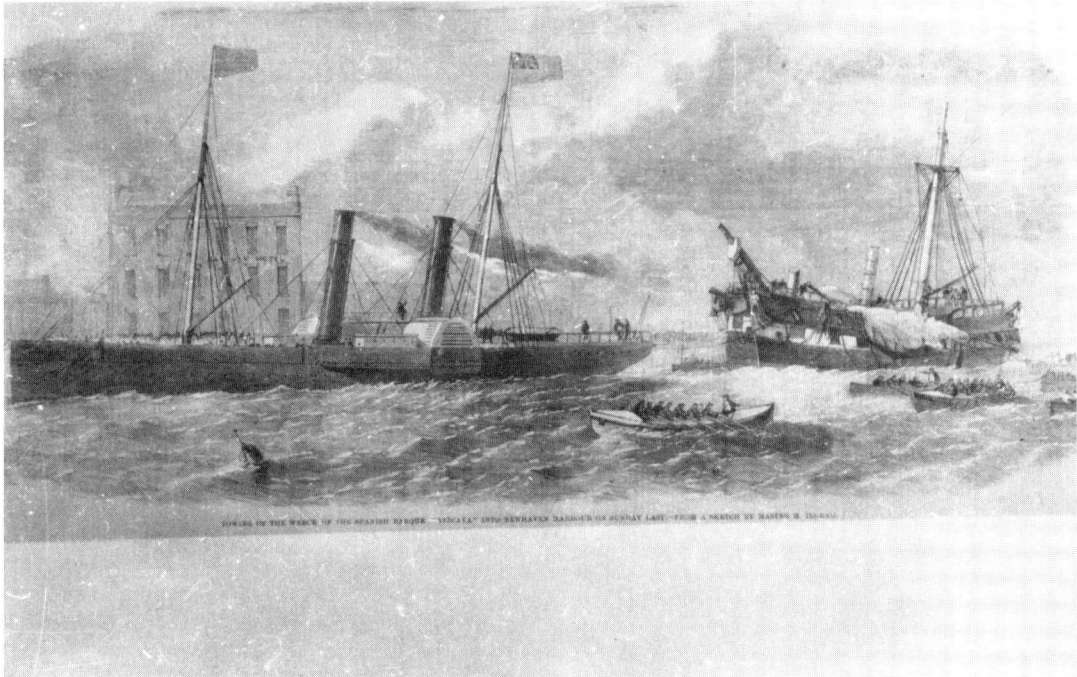

28. February 1859. The Spanish barque 'Vizcaya', run down by the Dutch ship 'D'Elmina' off Dungeness. She was intercepted off Rottingdean by the Newhaven steamer 'Lyon' and the Newhaven lifeboat 'Friend in Need'. The Admiralty Court awarded to the Newhaven steamer 'Lyon' the sum of £250 for bringing the wrecked vessel to harbour and to the crew of the lifeboat 'Friend in Need' the sum of £100.

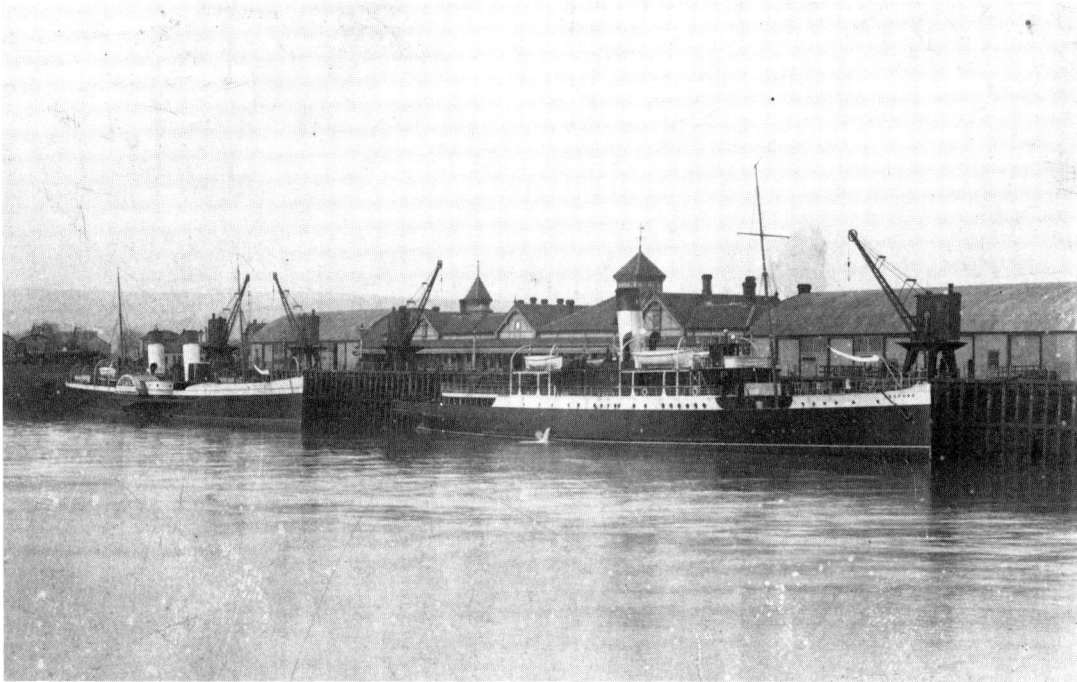

29. August 1895. The ill-fated 'Seaford' built in 1894. She was run down and sunk by the Newhaven cargo steamer 'Lyon' in 1895. A triple screw turbine steamer, 'Seaford', was reckoned to be one of the finest ships of the service. She was replaced by a sister ship 'Sussex'. 'Seaford' was one of the earliest 'screw' steamers in service.

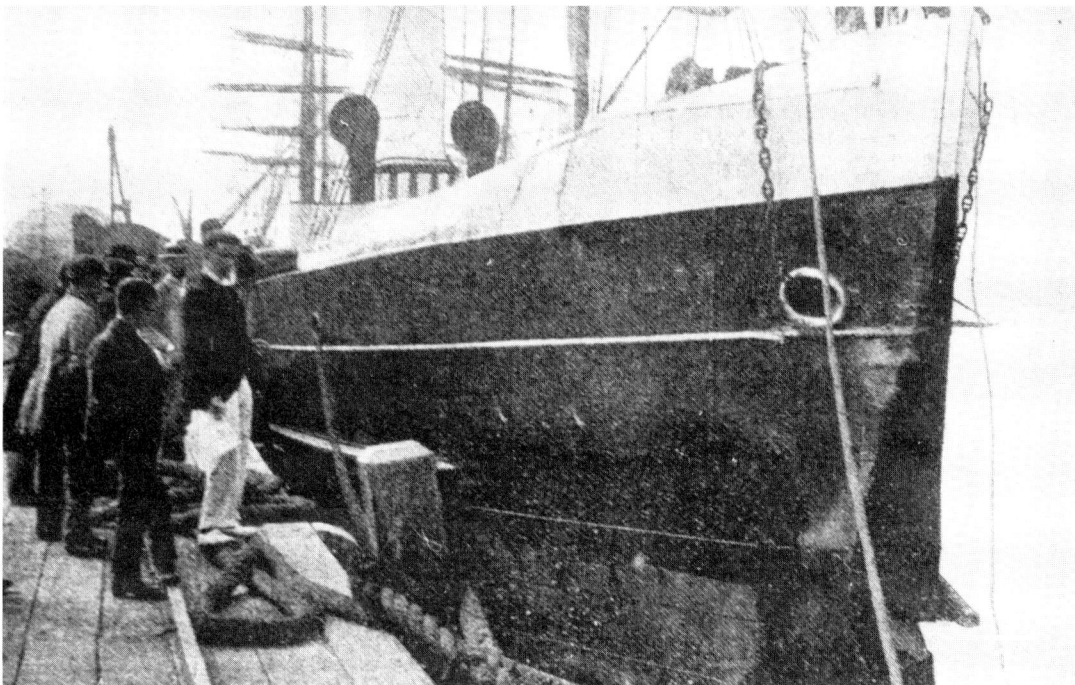

30. August 1895. This is the Newhaven steamer 'Lyon' with a badly damaged and crumpled bow, received when she ran down the new Newhaven/Dieppe mail boat 'Seaford' which was sunk, just one year old.

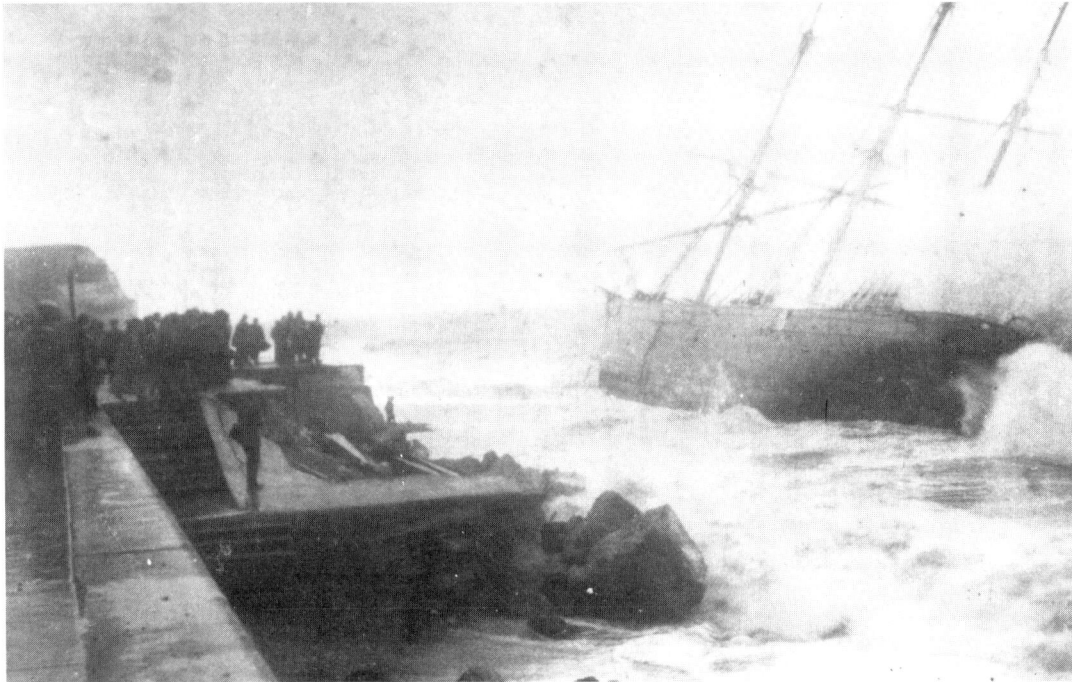

31. The fine sailing ship 'Peruvian' fetches up on the east beach just opposite the old 'Esplanade' hotel, 1899. The crew were taken off by the 'breeches' buoy' from Newhaven life saving unit. Two lives were lost. The Newhaven lifeboat 'Michael Henry III' was towed to the scene by the paddle tug 'Nelson' and the lifeboat, under command of coxswain George Winter, stood by. The 'Peruvian' was carrying a cargo of logwood and vegetable ivory, known locally as 'ivory nuts'. As 'Peruvian' broke up these nuts littered the beach and locals were paid something in the order of 2/- (10p) per cwt to recover them.

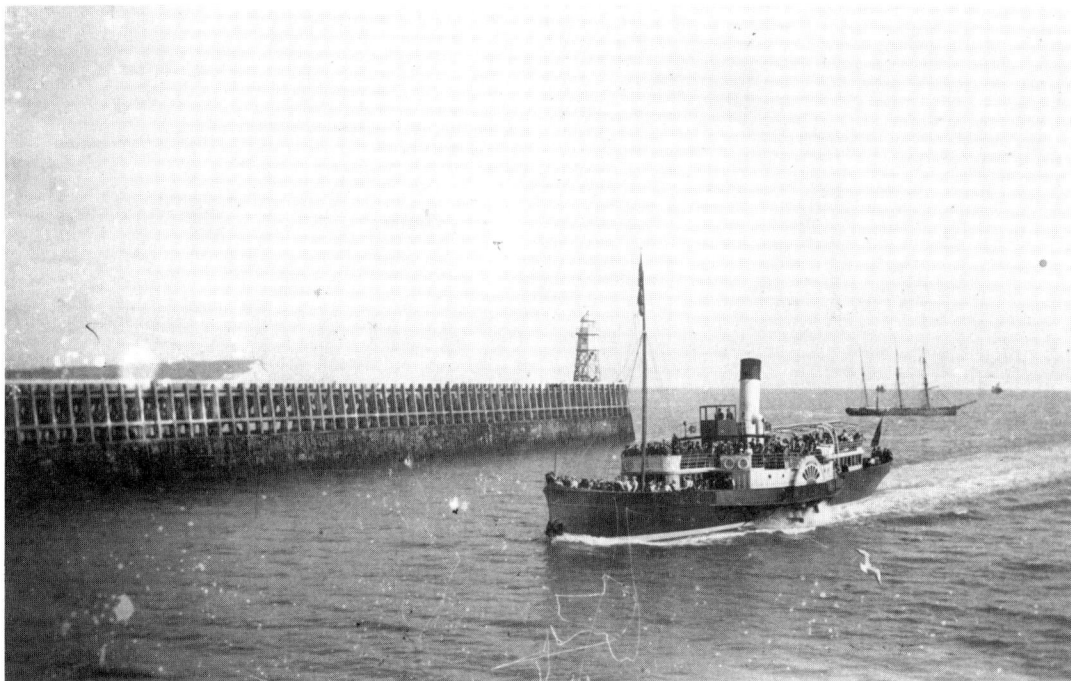

32. The year is 1899 — a heavily laden passenger excursion vessel calls into Newhaven harbour. The hundreds on board would not have wished for the fate of the boat in the background — she was the 'Oreala' carrying a load of stone, and sank within reach of the harbour.

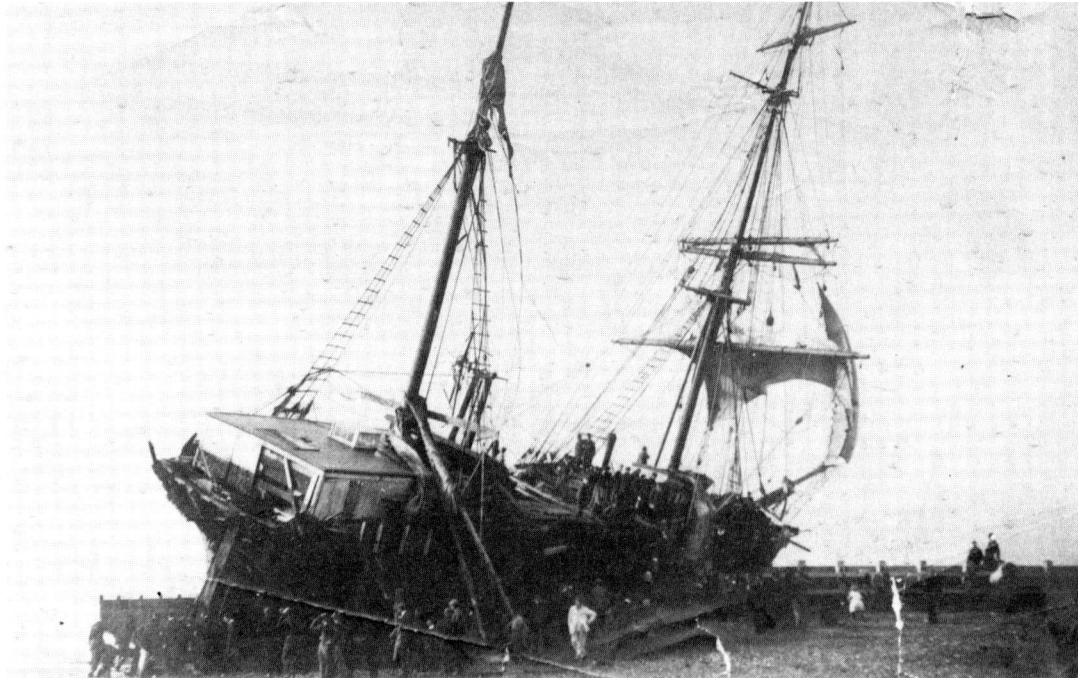

33. September 1900. The Norwegian sailing ship 'Sagaton' ran ashore on the east beach close to the Buckle Inn, Seaford. She was carrying a cargo mainly of oranges which found themselves all along the shoreline in a few days – a source of enjoyment for many!

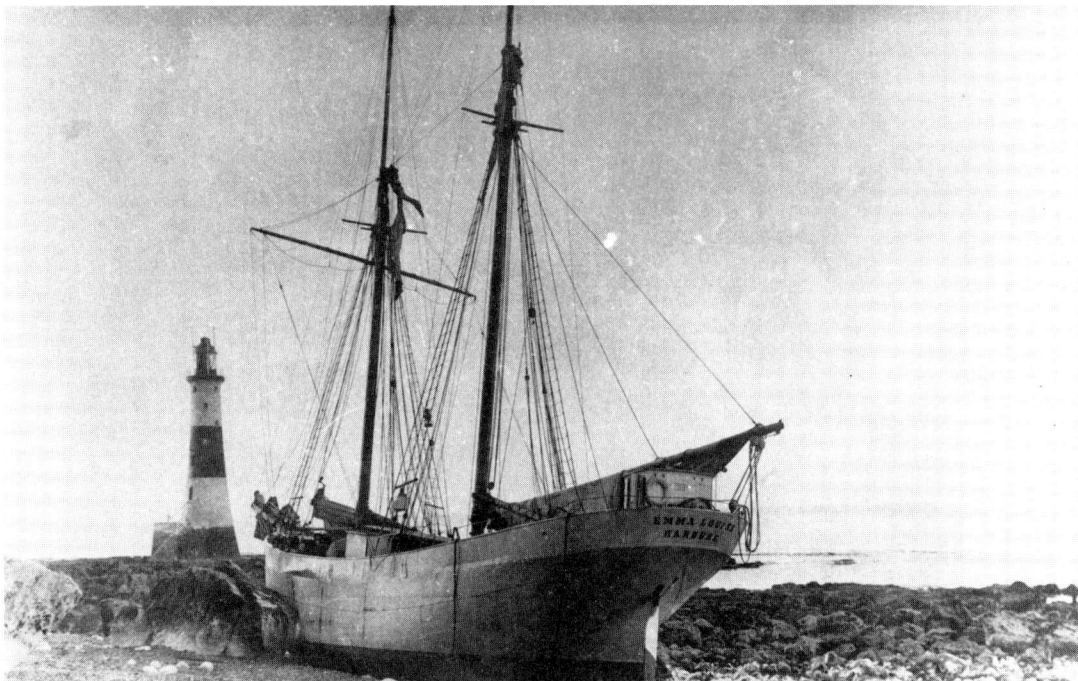

34. A coastal sailing vessel, 'Emma Louise' is seen here in 1906 ashore by Beachy Head lighthouse (they don't come much closer). She was carrying a cargo of china clay from the Cornish port of Charleston. Her crew were rescued by the Newhaven lifeboat 'Sir Fitzroy Clayton'.

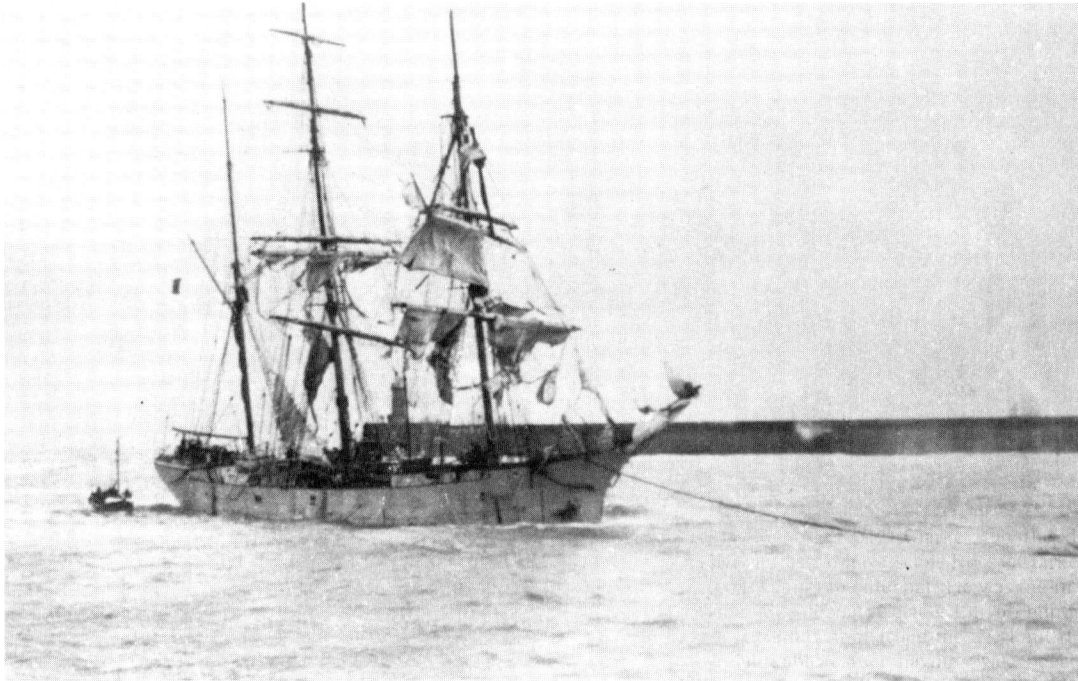

35. The Italian sailing ship 'Anirac' from Genoa experienced very heavy weather in the English channel losing most of her sails and deck cargo. 1906. She had to be helped into Newhaven harbour by the Shoreham tug 'Stella' and the lifeboat.

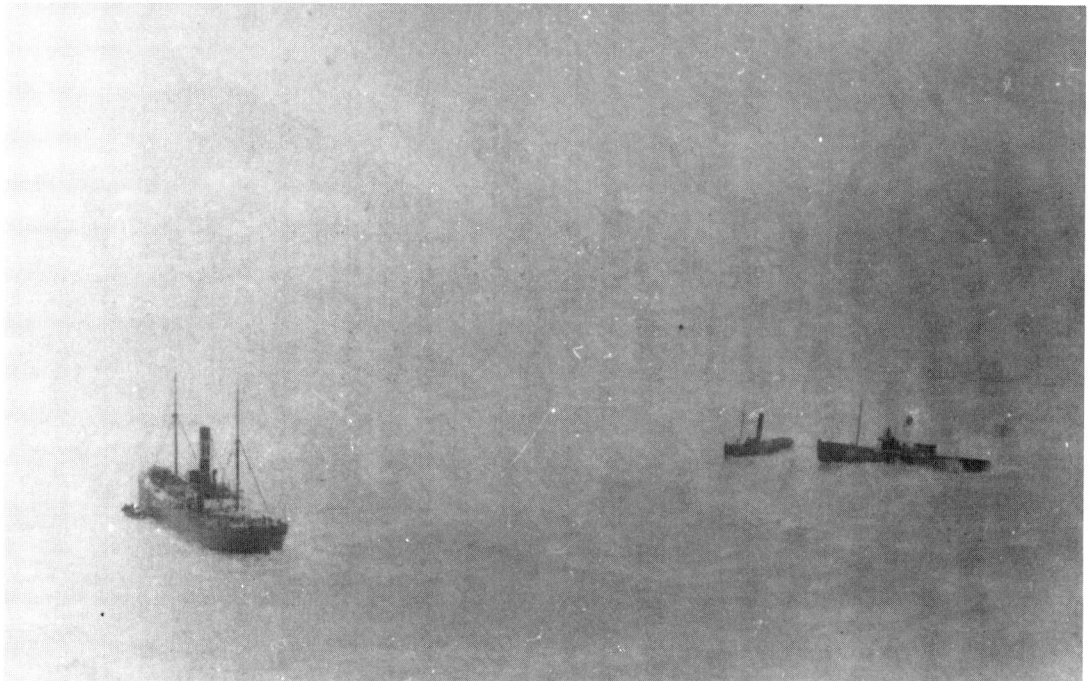

36. It was in March 1907 that the cargo steamer 'Newstead' ran aground at what locals call 'Puck Church parlour', at Seaford. She is seen with two tugs, 'Alert' and 'Belle of the Usk', together with the attendant lifeboat 'Michael Henry' standing by.

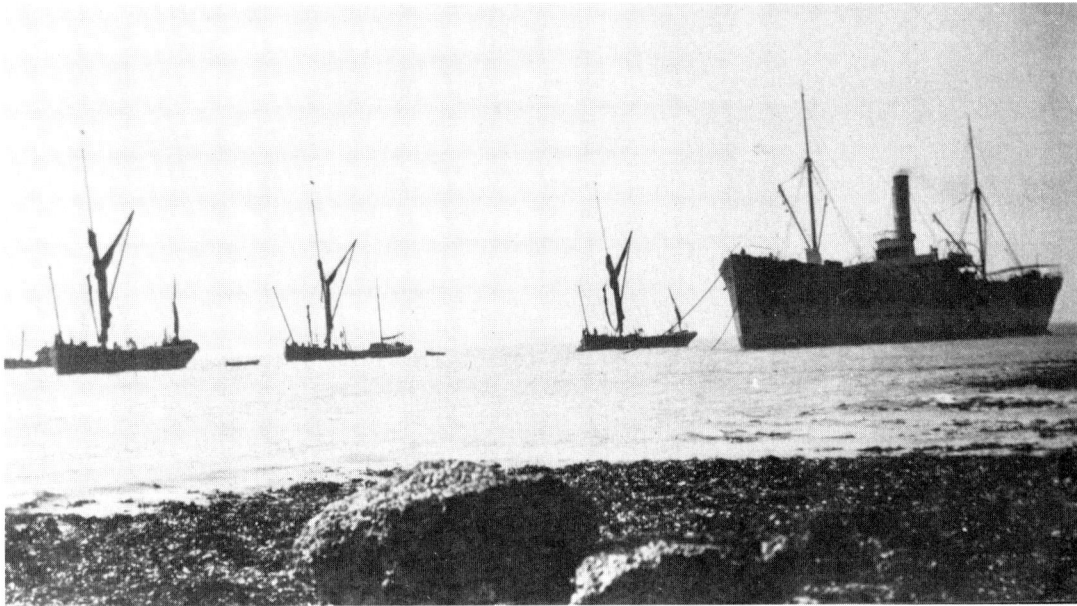

37. Before 'Newstead' could be floated off she had to be lightened and we see here barges offloading her cargo before eventually refloating.

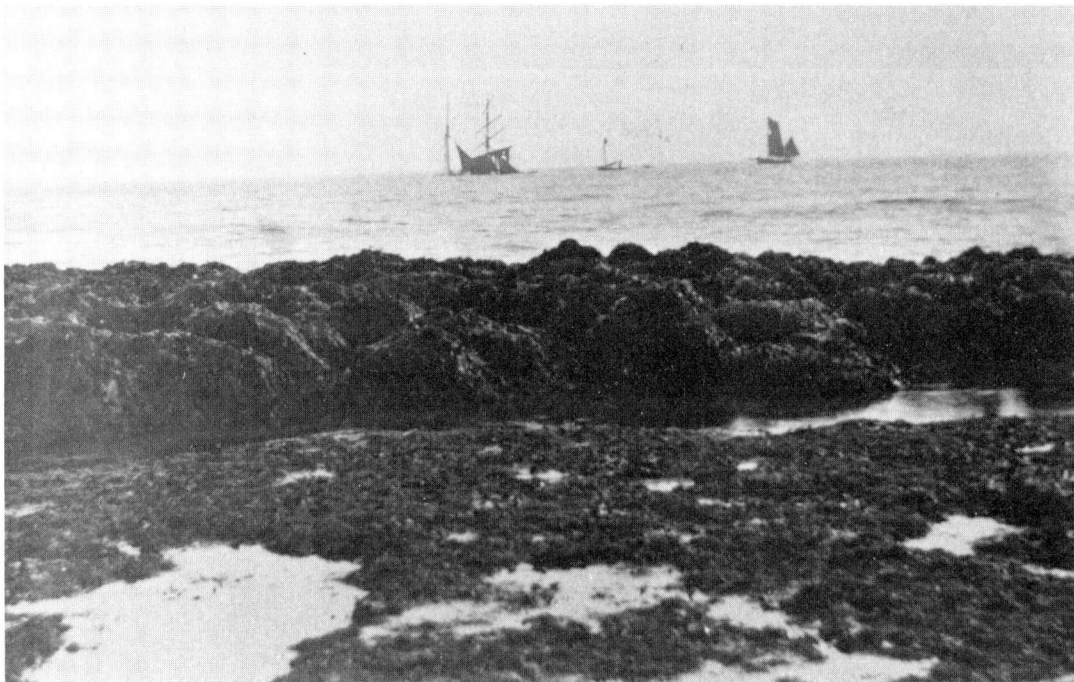

38. At the turn of the century there was still a preponderance of sail in coastal waters. Many small brigs, schooners etc. traded from Newhaven to the east coast coal ports and back as well as to Le Havre, Honfleur, Dieppe etc. Casualties were quite commonplace and as seen here many a ship was run down at night only to be discovered the following morning. This particular vessel was the brig 'Diadem' that had been run down by the steamer 'Hyndeford'.

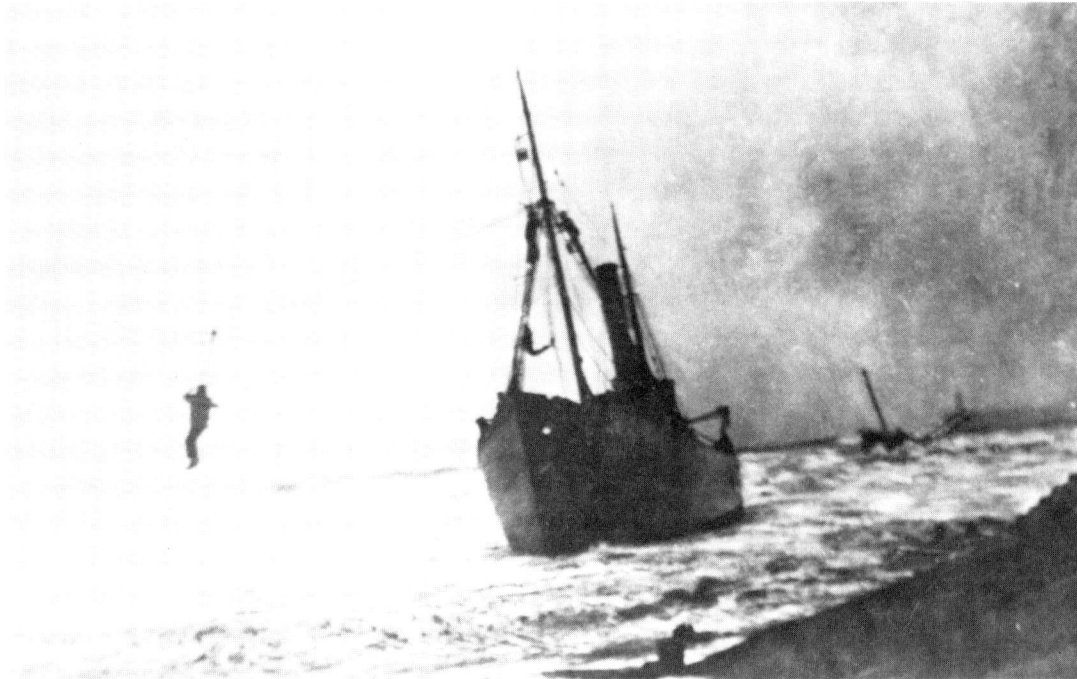

39. The trawler 'Gamecock' is — 1908 — seen ashore on the east beach by the 'Buckle', and this picture shews well the crew being taken off by breeches buoy. In the background we can see the Newhaven lifeboat 'Michael Henry IV' being rowed to the casualty.

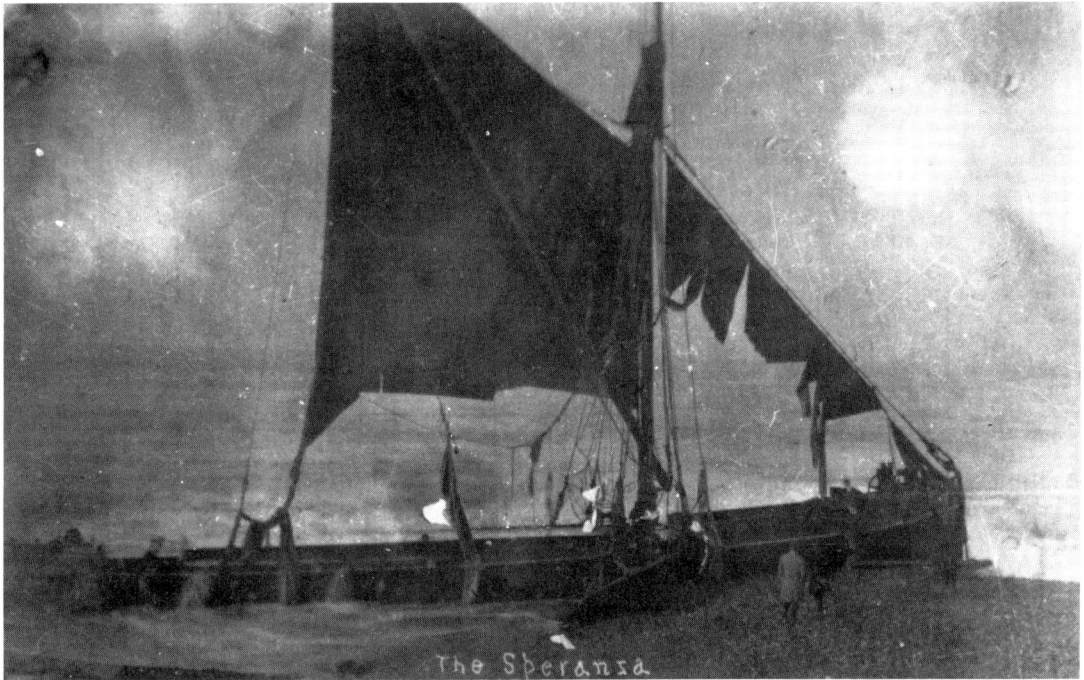

40. October 1911. A sailing barge, 'Speranza', grounds on the east beach by the Tidemills. This graphic illustration describes it all.

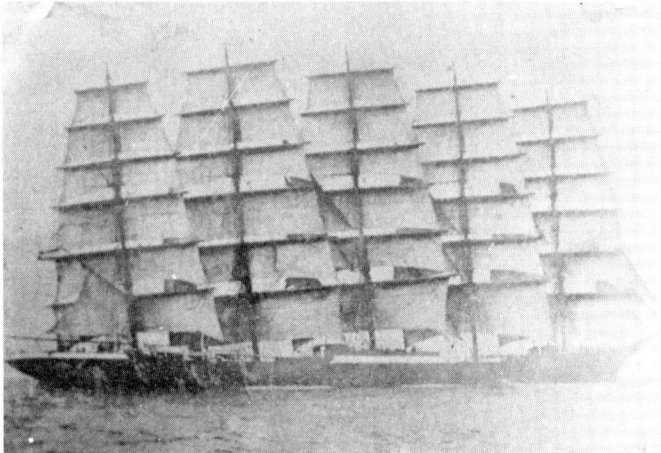

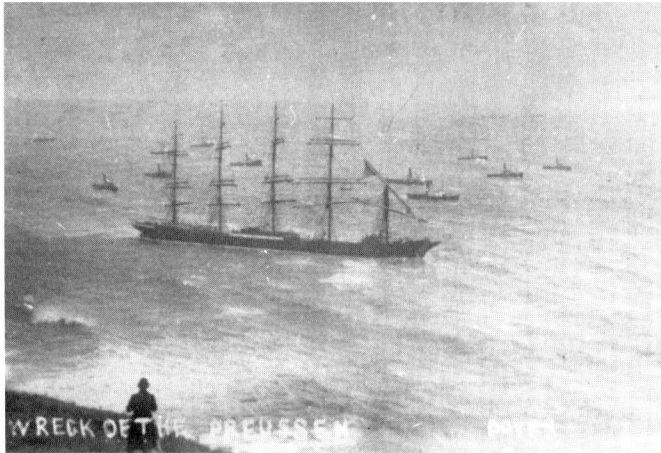

WRECK OF THE PREUSSEN

41. The mighty 'Preussen'. Here depicted is the worlds largest sailing ship (ship – square rigged on all masts). She was also the only 5 masted sailing ship in the world. Built in 1902 she was one of the famous 'Flying 'P' line of Germany. She displaced 11,150 tons! and could carry 8,000 tons of cargo. 490ft in length and 54ft beam with a draught of 27ft. She hauled 60,000 square feet of canvas. Her mainmast was 277ft high, she rigged 15 miles of wire, 10 miles of rope, 800 yards of cable and 1,260 blocks. She was run down off Newhaven by the mail boat 'Brighton IV' in 1911.

After the collision 'Preussen' went slowly about and made her way to Dover where she hoped to enter harbour. She ran aground in Crab Bay and although she eventually became a total loss every effort was made to save her and here we see some 12 tugs standing by hoping for the spoils of providence. 'Brighton' returned to Newhaven. A court of inquiry found that the British captain was at fault, the company was fined and the captain was dismissed the service. He later committed suicide.

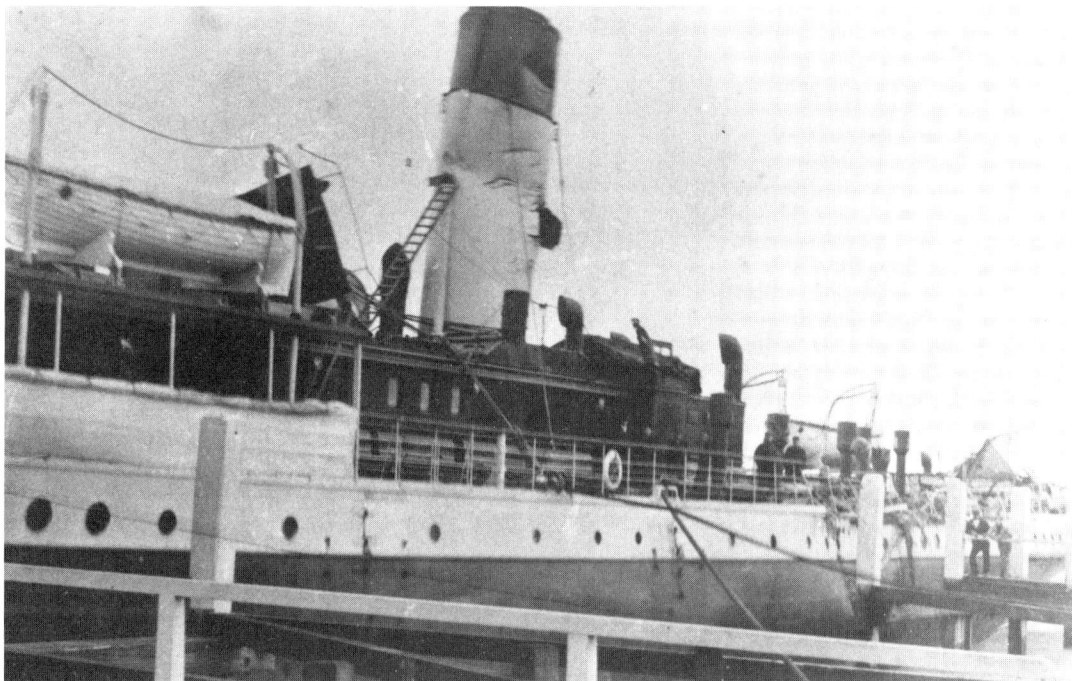

42. We saw earlier that 'Preussen' was the worlds largest sailing ship and one of the greatest of all the Cape Horners. On 5th November 1911, she was proceeding down channel to South America and at the same time 'Brighton IV' was leaving Newhaven for Dieppe on a cold foggy night. When she was first sighted by the night officer on 'Brighton' he misjudged her tremendous speed and attempted to cross her bow. The sailorman lost her bowsprit, most of her headgear on the foremast and badly sprung her stem, she could not steer as a result. 'Brighton' had her decks swept clear, she lost one funnell, a mast, lifeboats etc. The die was cast.

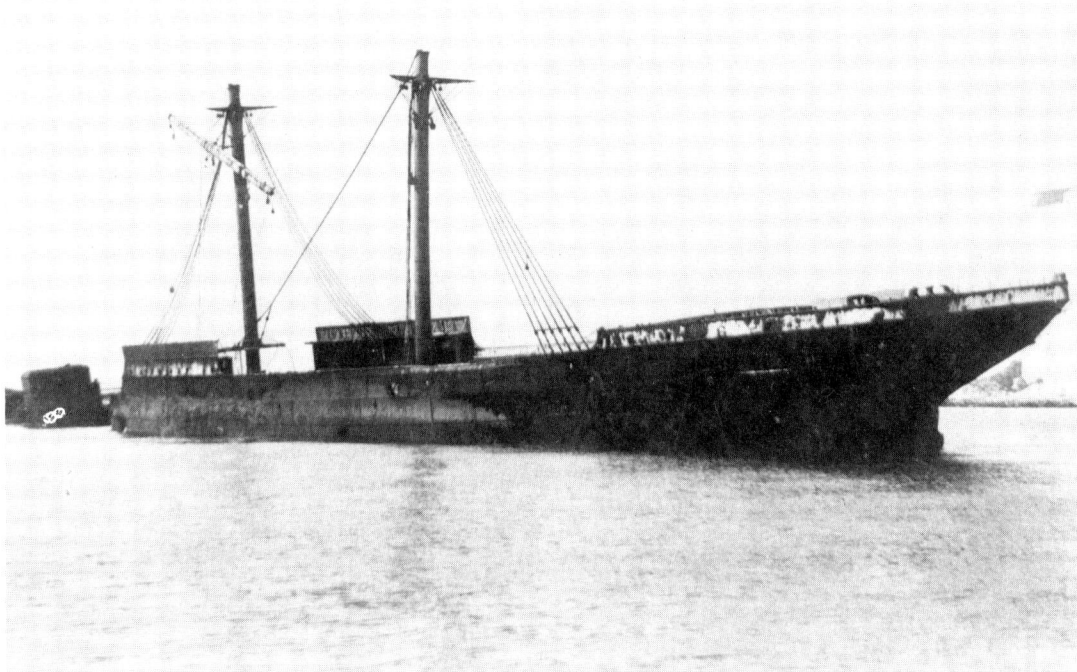

43. The last sigh... 'Preussen', the magnificent Queen of the sea, is doomed... She is badly breaking up and there is little to save. In later years – as now – at low tide her ribs can still be seen above the low water line.

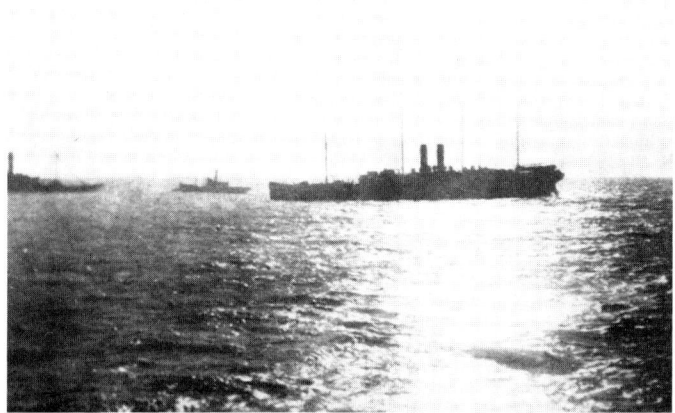

44. March 1912. The P & O Liner 'Oceana' on what was to have been her last trip to India is seen sinking by the bow after being run down by a four masted sailing ship 'Pisagua' – one of the famous flying 'P' line. The incident took place just off Beachy Head. She is seen here with the tug 'Alert' standing by as does the cargo vessel 'Garthmead'. 'Oceana' was carrying, as well as her passengers, a valuable cargo of 'bullion' all of which was salved by the Maritime Salvors vessel 'Ranger'.

March 1912. 'Oceana' incident. To think of a sailing ship running down a fine P & O Liner is hard indeed, but here we see the four masted barque 'Pisagua' which did just that. The 'Oceana' sank, but 'Pisagua' survived. She ran on down to Dover escorted by a local tug. The Newhaven lifeboat 'Michael Henry' went to assist and her crew were singled out for praise by the captain of the liner.

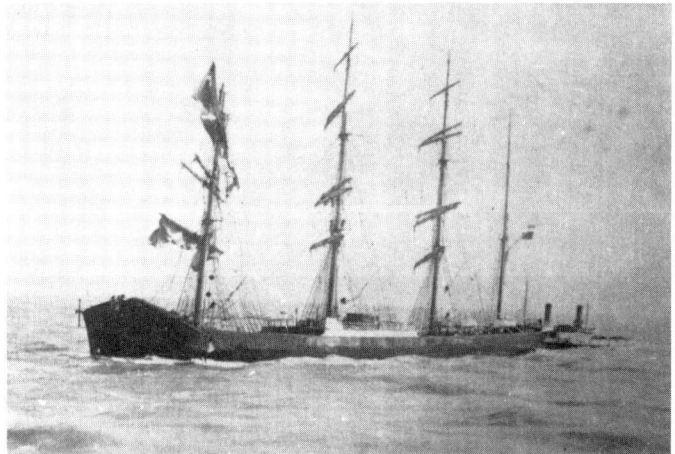

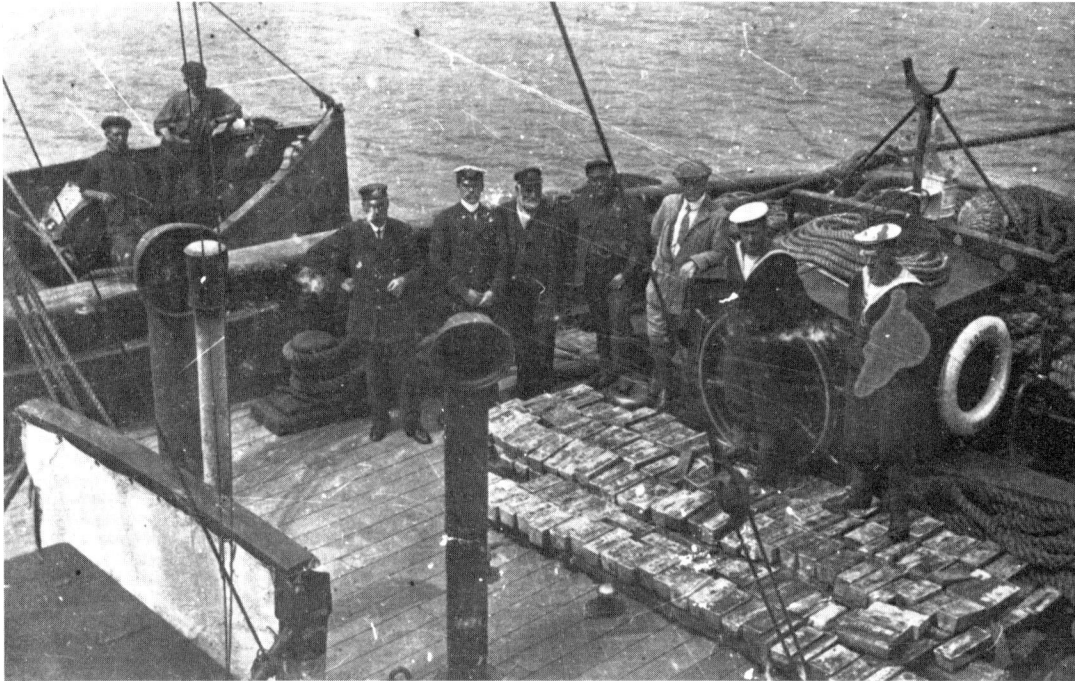

45. The 'Oceana' incident. As we have learned the 'Oceana' sank carrying several thousands of pounds worth of 'specie'. Here we see some of the recovered silver bars on the deck of the Newhaven based Maritime Salvors vessel 'Ranger'.

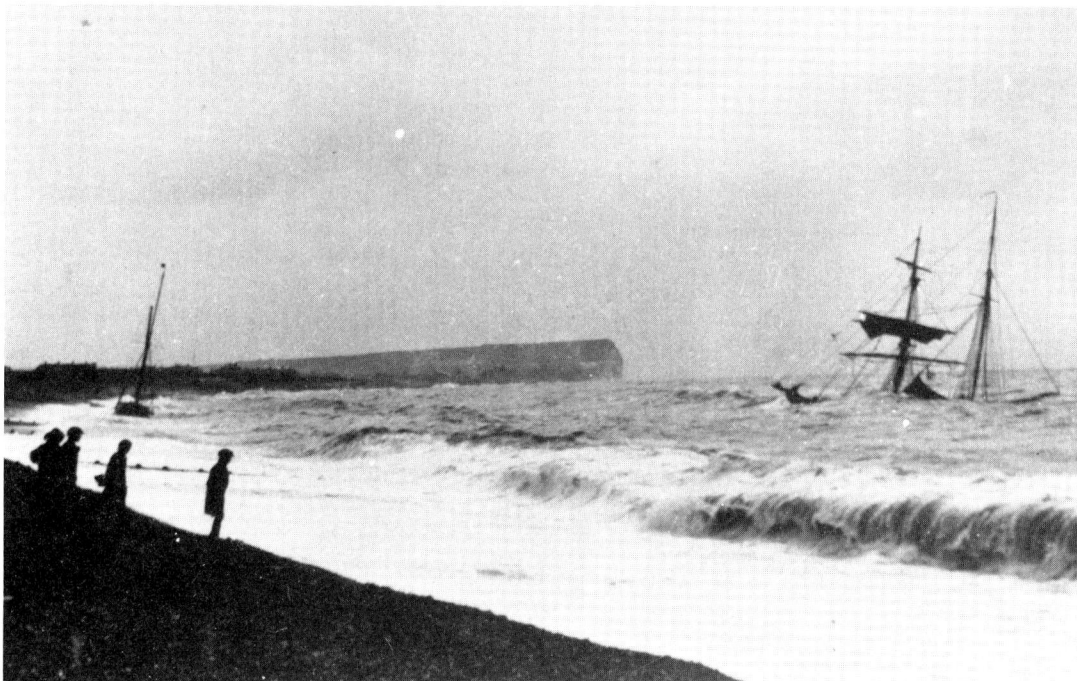

46. The barge 'Jachin' and the brig 'Catherine' both ran aground on the east beach, on 13th August 1914. Newhaven lifeboat 'Sir Fitzroy Clayton' took off the casualties. 'Catherine' became a total wreck whilst 'Jachin' was saved and still traded from Scandinavian ports well into the 1960s.

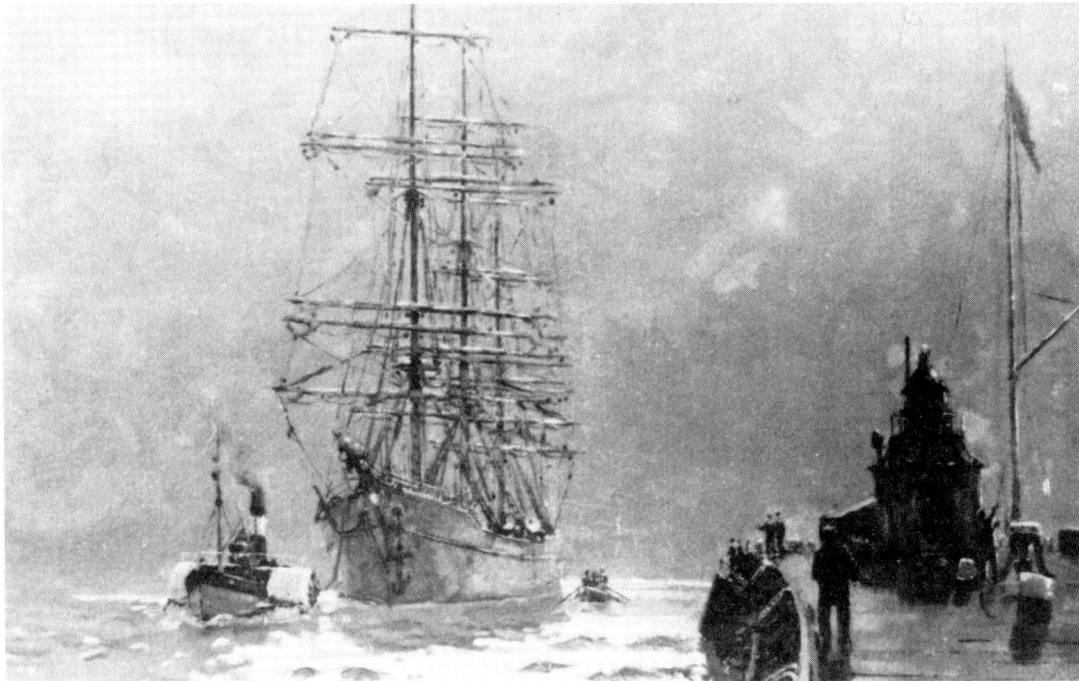

47. This very graphic picture I just call 'stormbound' − I think it says it all!

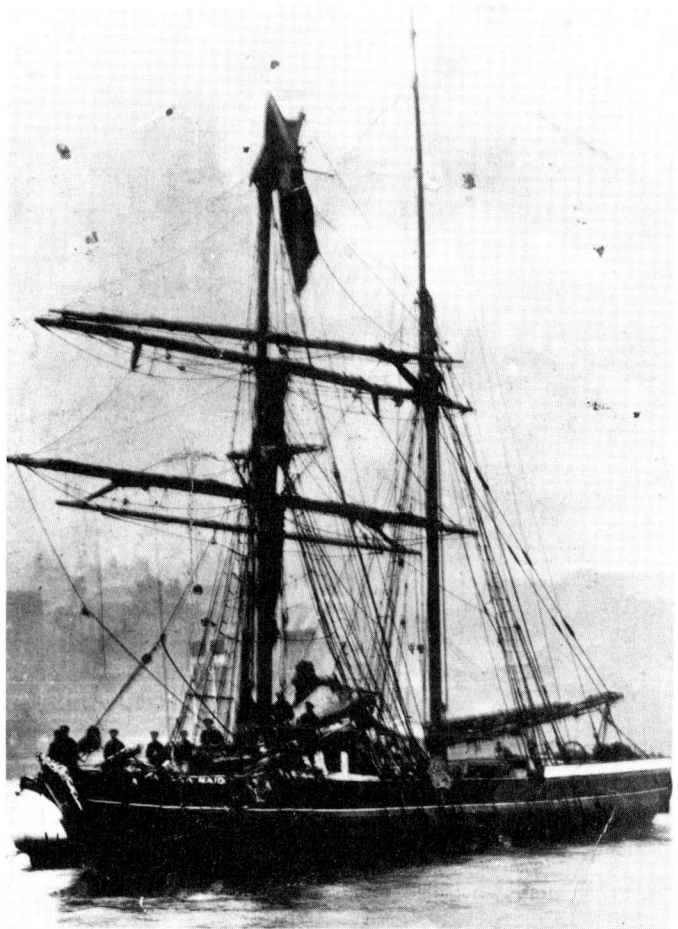

48. The coastal trader 'Sussex Maid' was one of many fine vessels built at Newhaven in John Grays shipyard. She is seen here suffering from storm damage to her 'tops' and foremast. She regularly brought coal to Newhaven from the east coast for the Gas Works Company.

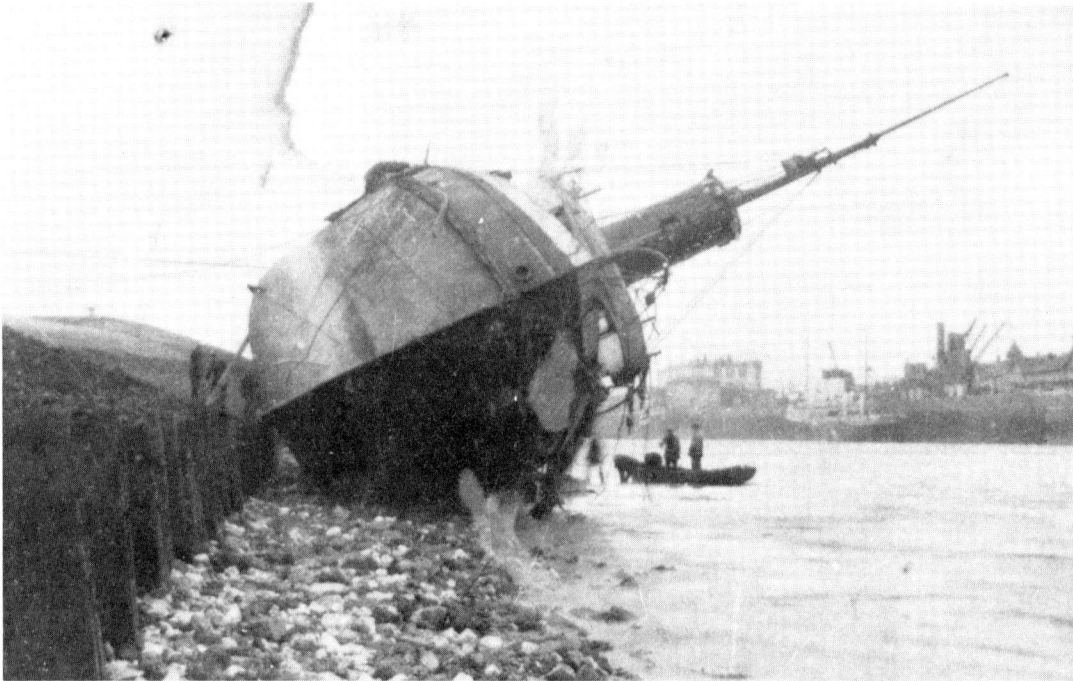

49. The little tug 'Gauntlett' was 1922 proceeding down river when her keel caught on the short piles of the harbour works and she stuck fast. As the tide receded she also went down, ever so slowly until she reached the position we see here. Skilful salvage works meant that all openings were plugged and a dredger was made fast alongside and she slowly righted herself on the next tide.

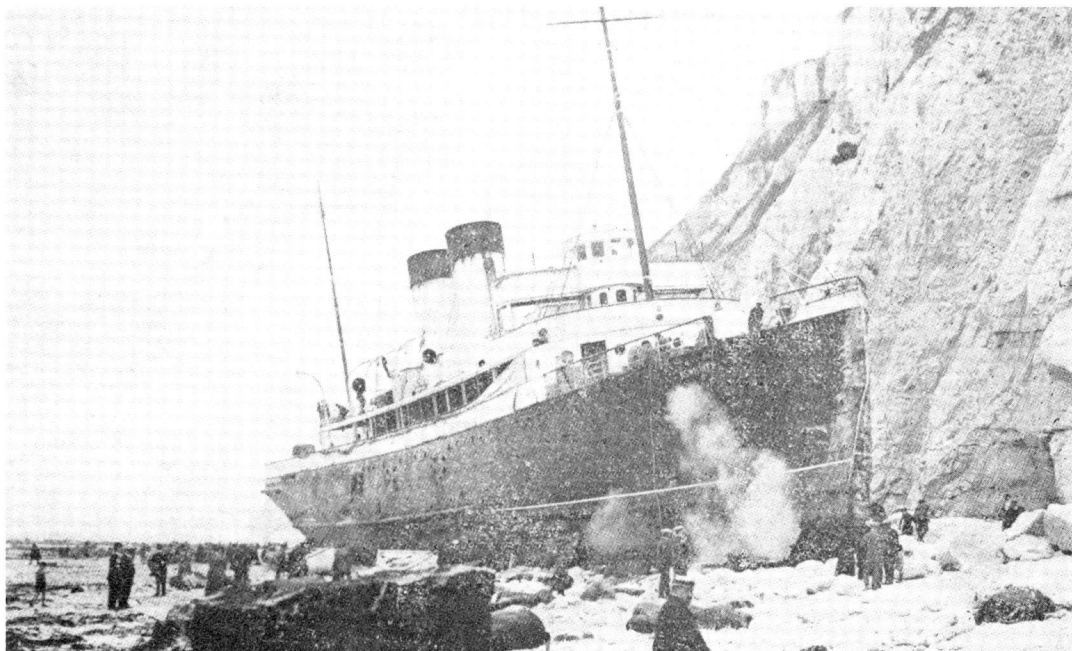

DIEPPE. 5 AOUT 1924. - Le Paquebot "Newhaven" échoué sur la Côte de Berneval   Imp.-Pap. L. VIDIÈRE. — Di

50. August 1924. The Newhaven/Dieppe service mail boat 'Newhaven' got into difficulties on the approach to Dieppe and she foundered on the rocks at Berneval. Apart from damage to her bow and some damage to the deck caused by falling rocks she was little damaged and soon returned to service. 'Newhaven' survived the war and returned to service at the termination of hostilities – little changed, except that she had then only one funnel.

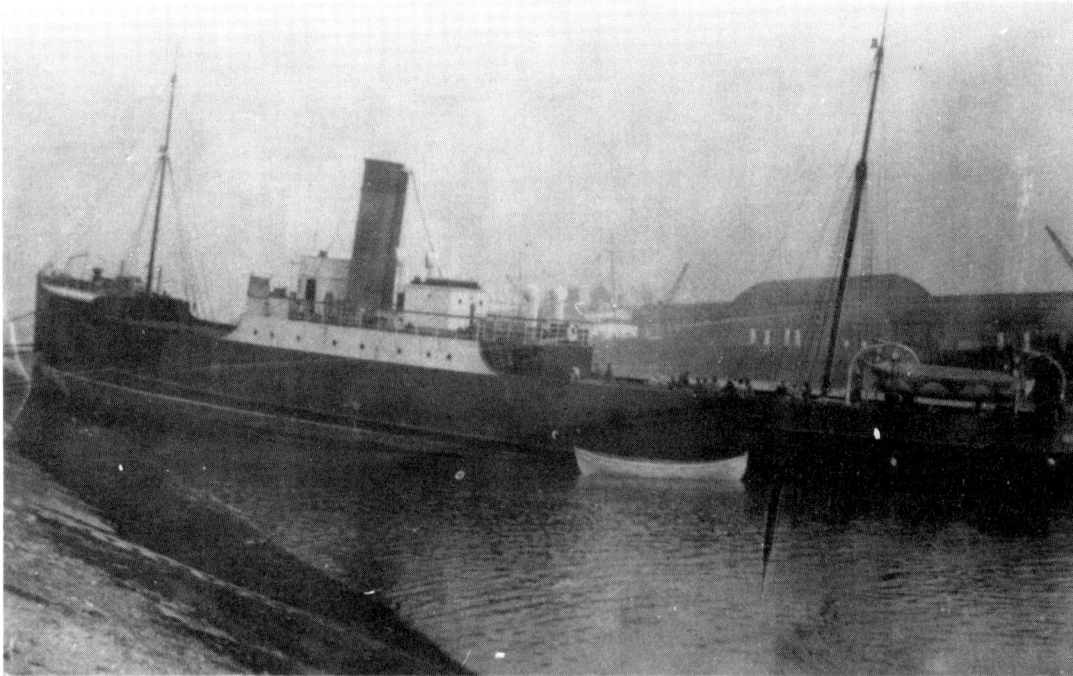

51. Even in the best of circumstances and regulated conditions things can go wrong with a capital 'W'. On 2nd January 1927 the Newhaven/Dieppe service cargo vessel 'Rennes' ran up the bank by the 'green light' right inside the harbour. She suffered little damage – a little bit of hurt 'dignity' no doubt.

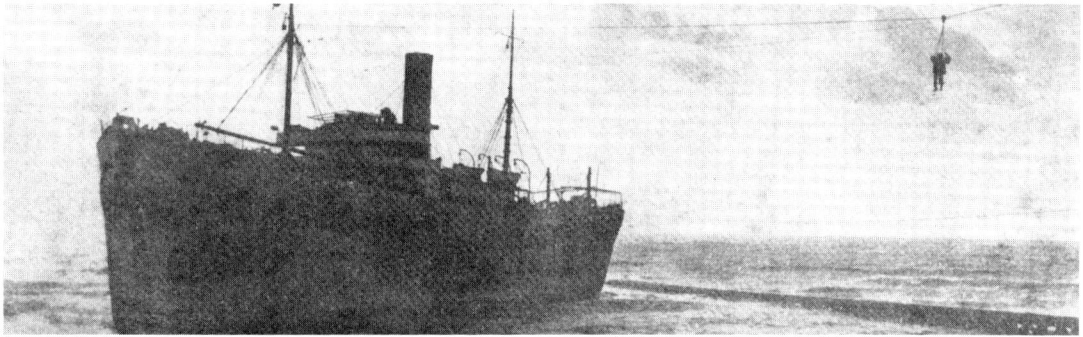

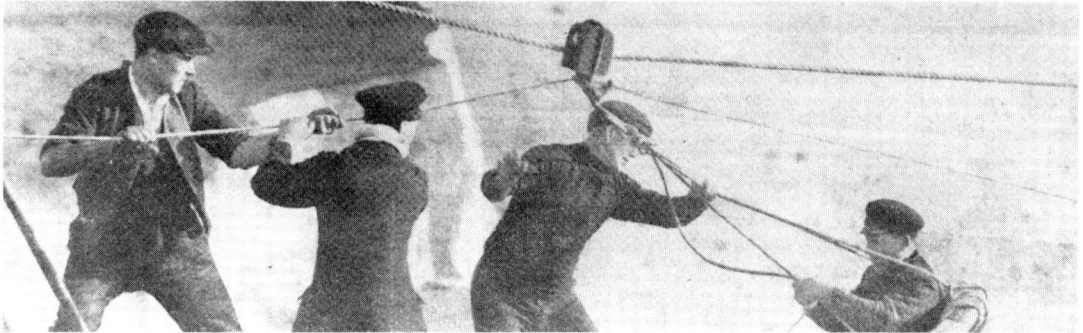

52. November 1929. During the night of 11th November 1929 the Italian cargo ship 'Nimbo' was proceeding down channel in a southerly gale when she ran aground on the outfall at Portobello, Telscombe Cliffs. Due to her precarious position and the gale force winds it was decided to take off the crew to the clifftop by the breeches buoy and the Newhaven crew under command of Mr. Vacher took off the crew of twenty without injury.

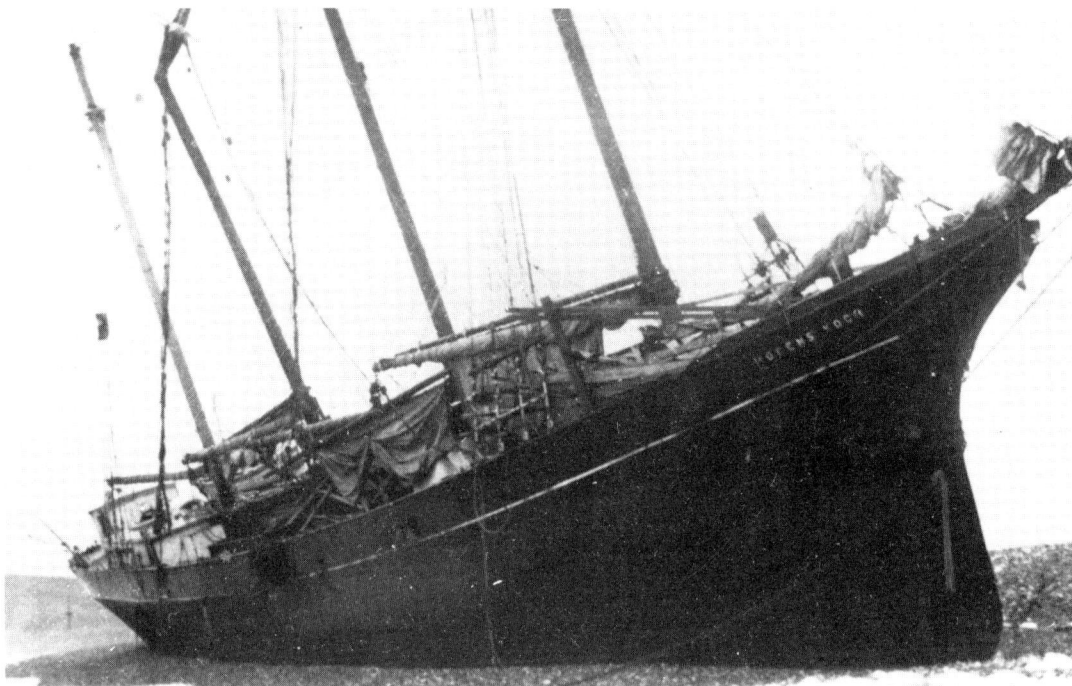

53. December 1929. Newhaven experienced the highest wind speeds since records were kept − gusting up to 112 miles per hour. The Danish four masted motor schooner 'Mogens Koch' got into difficulties and foundered at Cuckmere Haven. The Newhaven lifeboat 'Sir Fitzroy Clayton' received her second call for help that day and set out on an epic service. It took several hours to make the short journey to Cuckmere due to the severe winds, but they made it successfully and took off the crew of ten after several attempts. It was on the way back that they nearly met disaster whilst crossing the bay. A huge sea crashed into the boat and it all but sank − every one on board was injured, coxswain Payne received a broken pelvis, an injury from which he never recovered.

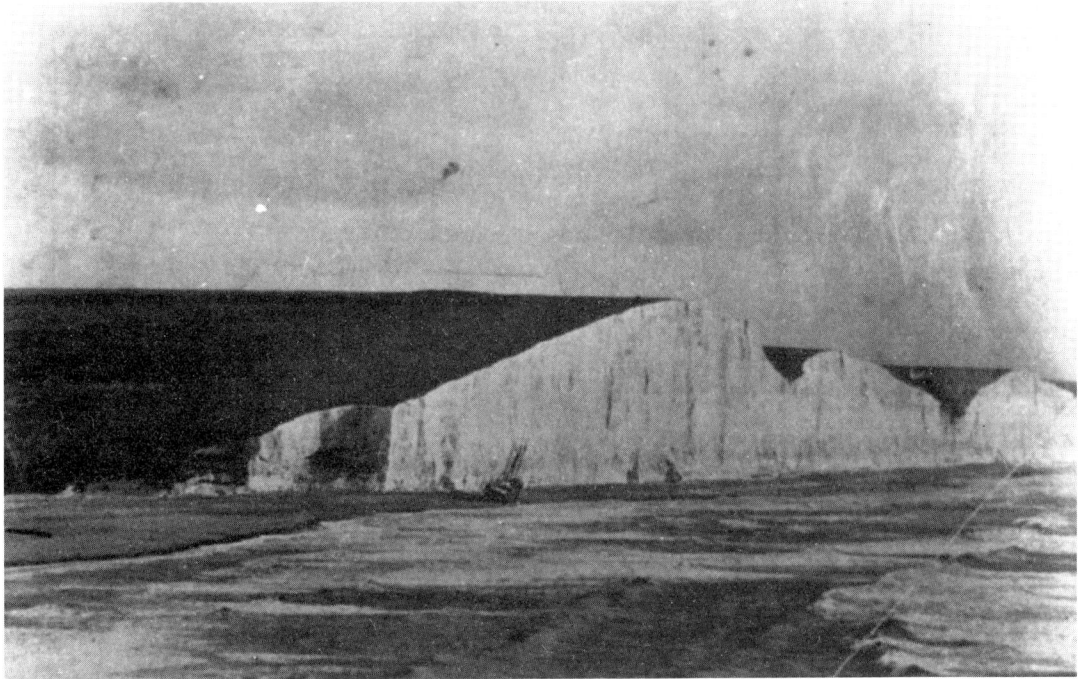

54. With the passage of just a few hours the wind has abated and the sea has dropped. 'Mogens Koch' sits forlornly on the shore prior to being refloated and taken to Newhaven. The King of Denmark said that the rescue of his countrymen had sent a wave of enthusiasm through his country.

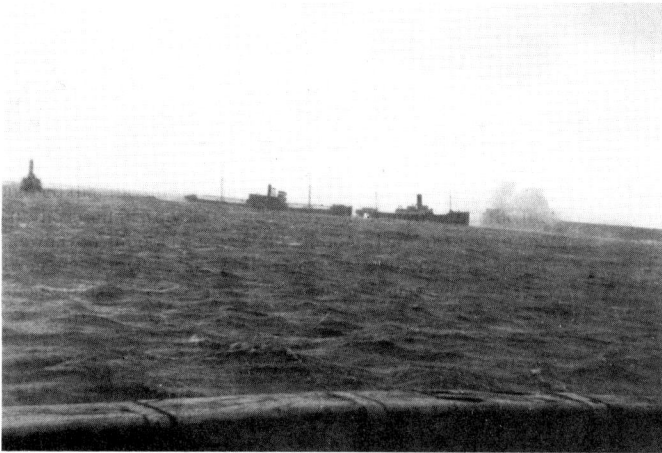

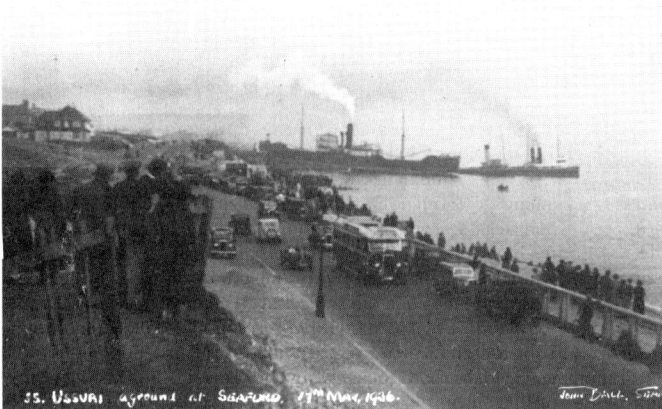

55. Ussuri aground at Seaford, 17th May, 1936.   John Bull, Seaford

55. September 1930. A large cargo ship, 'Peter Benoit', with a damaged rudder lies helpless in the bight of the breakwater in a very rough sea. The Newhaven tug 'Foremost 22' comes down out of the wind to assist. The Newhaven/Dieppe cargo ship 'Rennes' stands by to assist if required.

17th May 1936. The Russian steamer 'Ussuri' ran aground at Seaford east beach in spectacular style running almost onto the main coast road itself. Whilst local tugs 'Foremost 22' and 'Lady Brassey' stood by throughout the incident the master of 'Ussuri' refused all aid preferring to wait for the arrival of another Russian vessel to get her off. All in all it was a 'big' day out for the family.

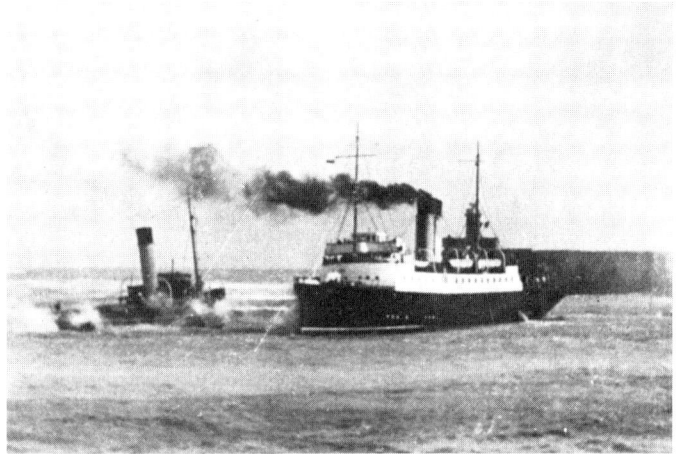

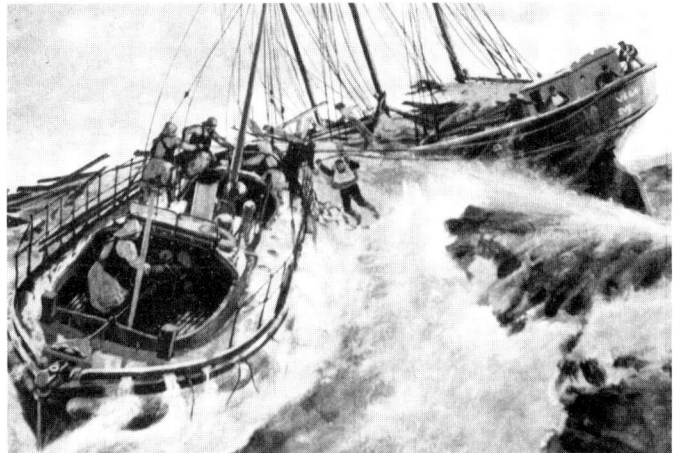

56. Until the advent of modern 'bow thrusters' and more powerful engines this was not an uncommon sight at Newhaven. Ships rounding the breakwater in high winds would often find themselves stuck fast on the sand bar and having to seek help. Here, the Newhaven mail boat 'Rouen' is in just such a situation and the tug 'Foremost 22' went to her aid. Even in the 1930s, ultra modern steamers on the service would carry a foresail to give stability rounding the breakwater.

November 1954. The Dutch schooner 'Vega' was abandoned off Beachy Head. HMS 'Vigo' stood by the three masted wooden vessel which was carrying timber to Shoreham. Her crew later rejoined her in Sheerness after having recovered at Newhaven. On 26th November the crew radio'd that she was taking in water. Newhaven lifeboat 'Cecil & Lilian Philpott' launched and stood by. Conditions deteriorated and coxswain Bill Harvey, being conscious of the moving deck cargo, decided to take off the crew by 'breeches buoy'. He later received the Institutions silver medal as well as the 'Maude Smith' award.

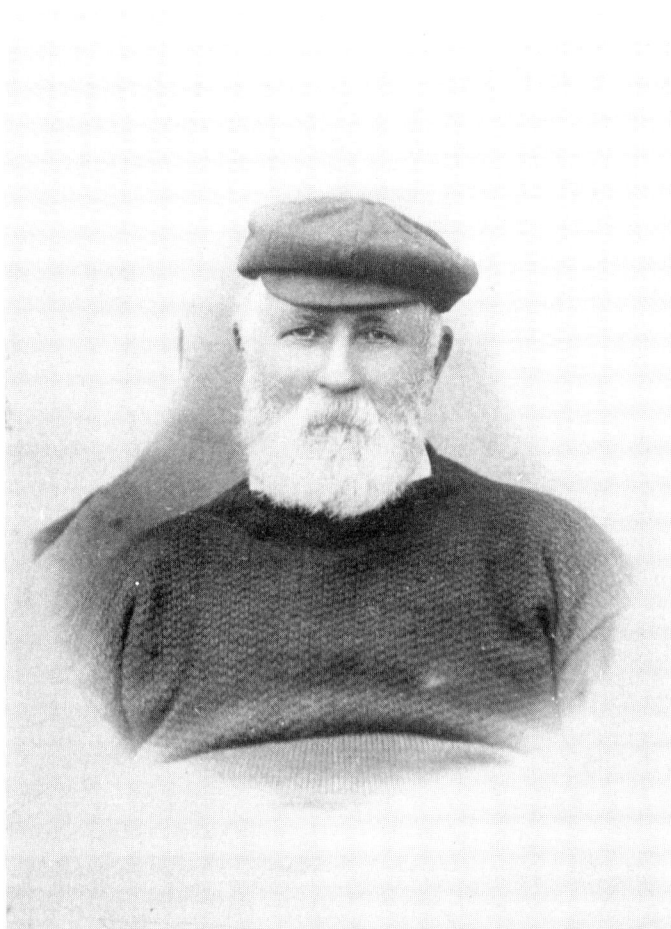

57. Coxswain Lower about 1881. Coxswain of the Newhaven lifeboat 'Michael Henry II' he came from a long line of seafarers. His grandson Dick Lower went to sea on the old 'Sir Fitzroy Clayton' lifeboat back with my grandfather. The family became one of Newhaven's foremost shipbuilders in the same stamp as 'Ernire' Cantell. I – the chronicler – was proud to have called 'Dick' Lower one of my friends.

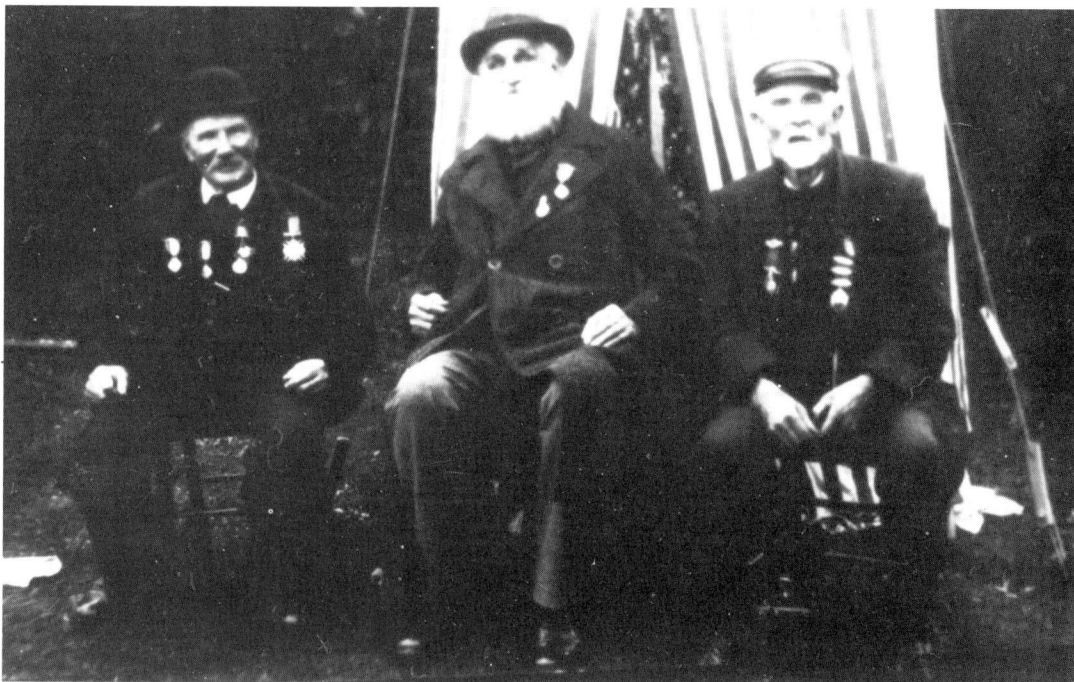

58. Three 'Worthies' of Newhaven — in more ways than one. Pictured here are three great lifeboatmen of the very early days of the Newhaven Station. From left to right we see 'Tucker' Winder, 'Dick' Winter and 'Ned' Holland. Dick Winter was, as was his brother George, coxswain of Newhaven lifeboats. They were both 'giants' of men in more than just stature.

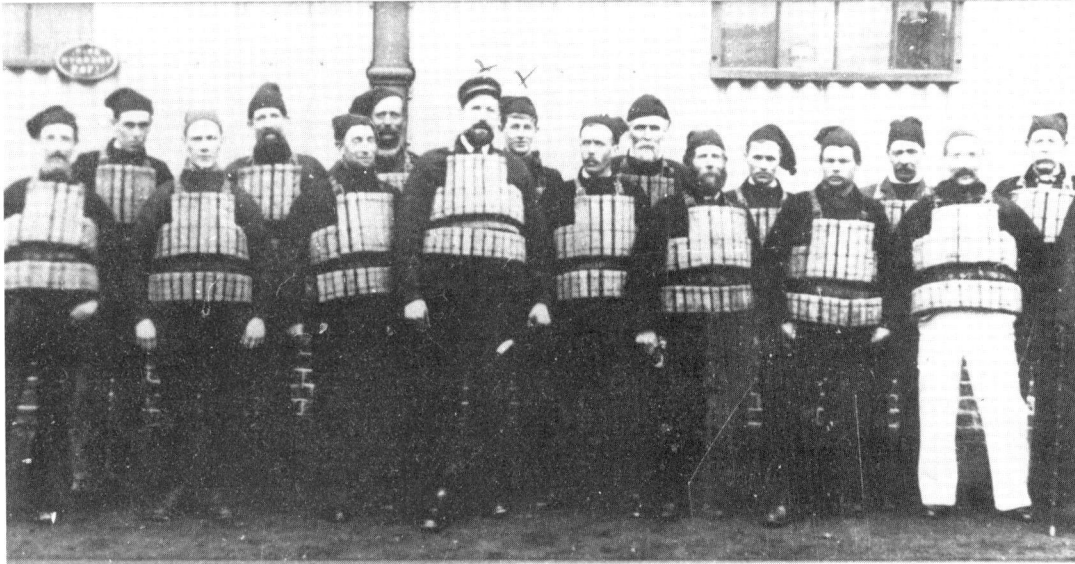

59. Here we see a fine body of men... the days of wooden ships and iron men. This is the crew of the lifeboat 'Michael Henry III' taken in the late 1890s. The crew still wore cork lifejackets and there is no doubt that the later 'kapock' lifejackets made movement much more easy. There is a very obvious age difference between members.

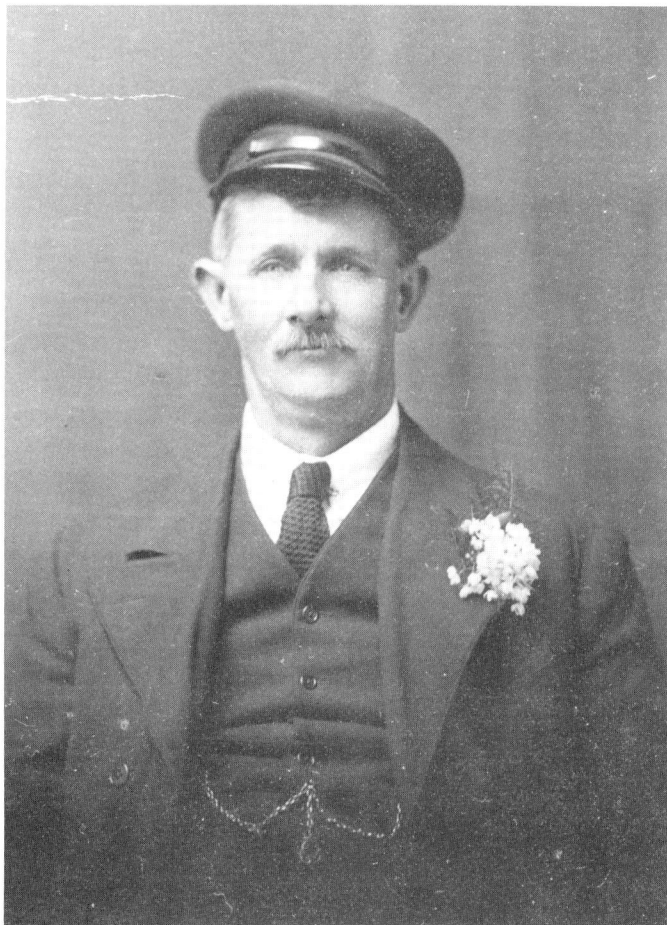

60. Coxswain Ricard 'Dick' Payne joined the lifeboat about 1889. He became bowman in 1908, second coxswain 1911 and coxswain in 1913. He died as a result of the serious injuries he received whilst on service to the rescue of the Danish motor schooner 'Mogens Koch' in December 1929. He was the holder of the Institution Bronze and Silver Medals as well as the Maude Smith award for the bravest act of lifesaving in 1924. The King of Denmarks' representative in London presented him with a solid gold full hunter watch. The family have over 100 years of unbroken service on the Newhaven lifeboats.

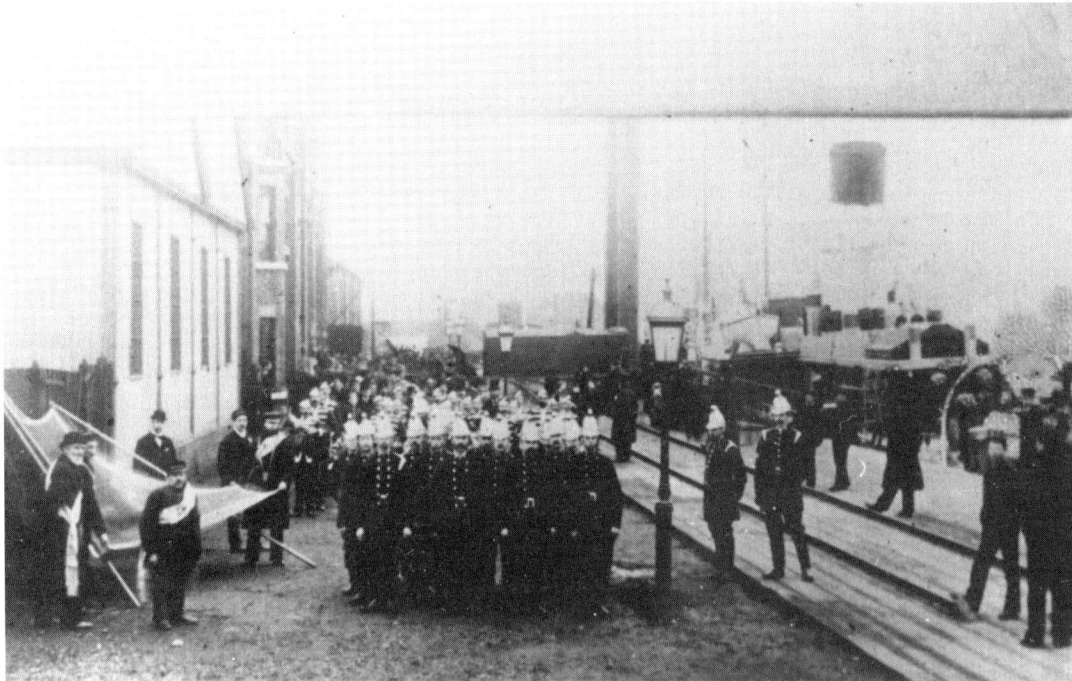

61. Fete day at Newhaven. Outside of the Marine workshops are lined up the local Fire Brigade Band, the lifeboat crew and other notables just about to set off through the town fund raising and generally 'shewing the flag'.

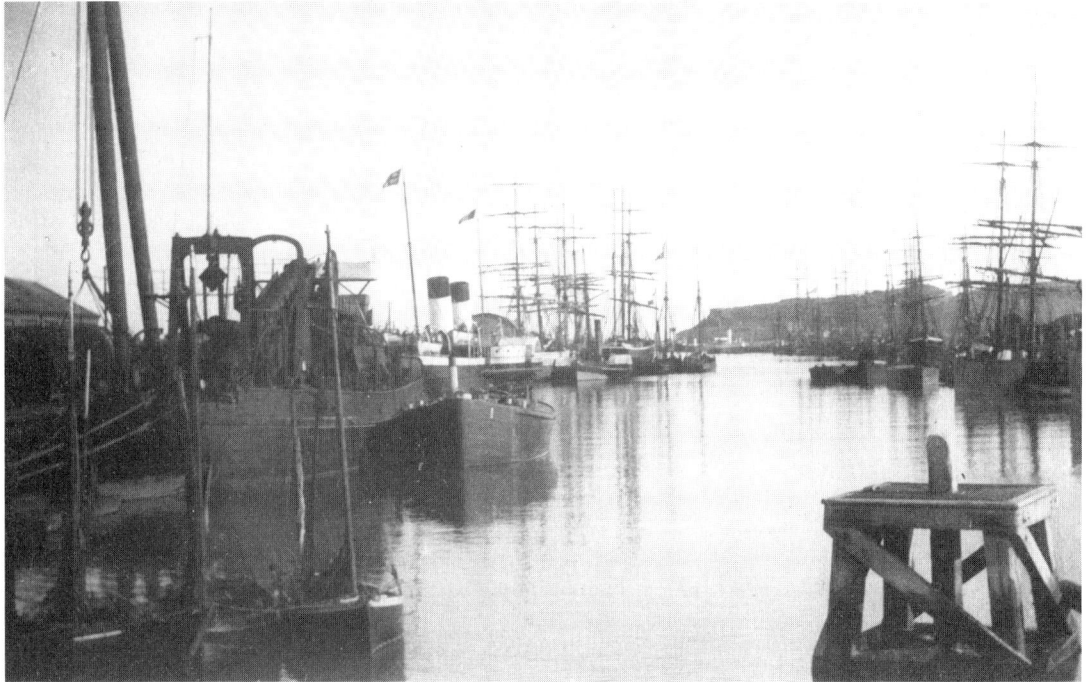

62. In the 1890s Newhaven was classified as the sixth most important port in the kingdom, quite an achievement for a small town. Under the expert guidance and control of the London Brighton South Coast Railway Co., in partnership with the Western Co. of France, they ran services not only to Dieppe, but to Honfleur, Caen, Fecamp, the Mediteranean, the Baltics and South America. This 1896 photograph shows the large number of sailing vessels in the harbour, all being grateful that there was always available a modern well-crewed lifeboat.

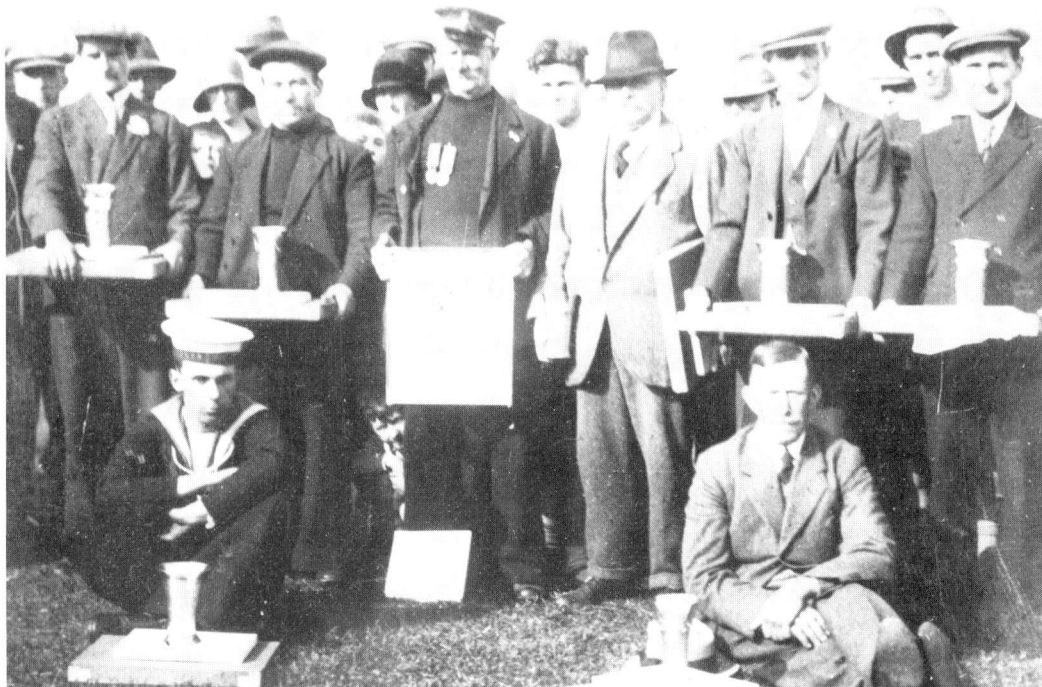

63. An award presentation ceremony at the recreation ground, Newhaven, in 1930, after the epic rescue of the crew of ten of the Danish vessel 'Mogens Koch'. The King of Denmark gave awards to every crew member in the shape of silver goblets with a solid gold full Hunter watch being given to the coxswain, suitably inscribed – of course.

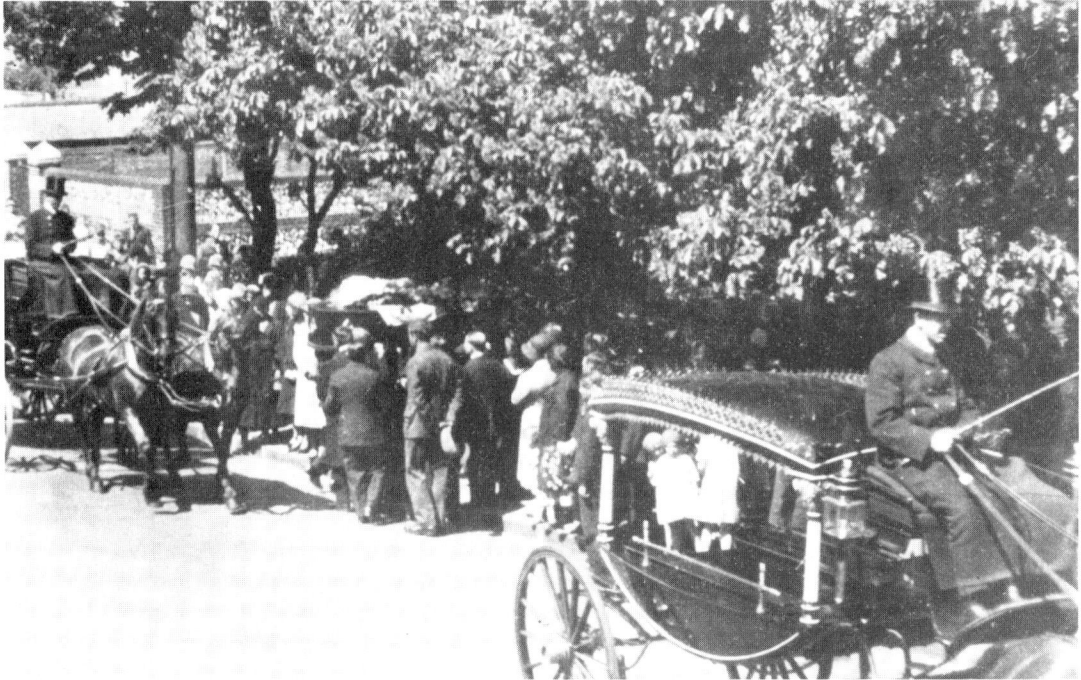

64. Impressive scens witness the funeral of the late coxswain Ricard 'Dick' Payne, long serving lifeboat-man and resident of Newhaven. He died at the age of 57 as a result of the serious injuries he received whilst on service to the rescue of the crew of ten of the Danish motor vessel 'Mogens Koch'. He was succeeded as coxswain by his lifetime friend and shipmate Willie 'Rocky' Clarke.

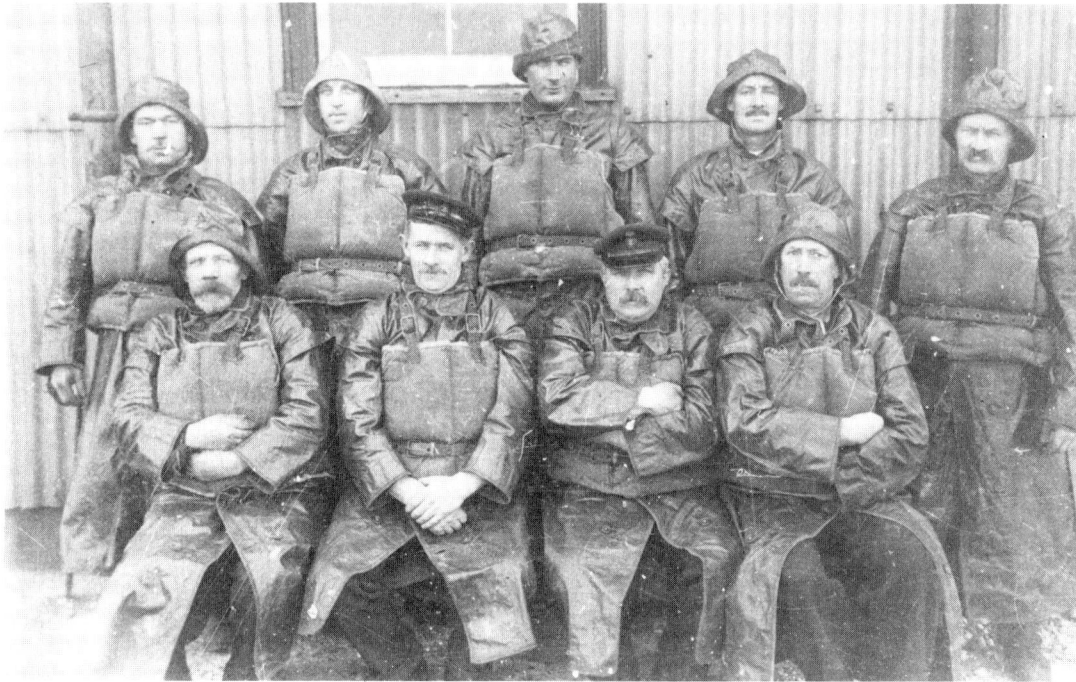

65. This crew photograph of the 'Sir Fitzroy Clayton' lifeboat was taken outside of the harbour masters boathouse. We see here 'Buff' Jones, Jack Clarke, George Winder, George Parker, 'Dabbler' Fred Payne, 'Rocky Clarke', 'Dick' Payne, Ernie Cantell and Fred Parker. These were the men that so valiantly served not only the boat but also the town and harbour.

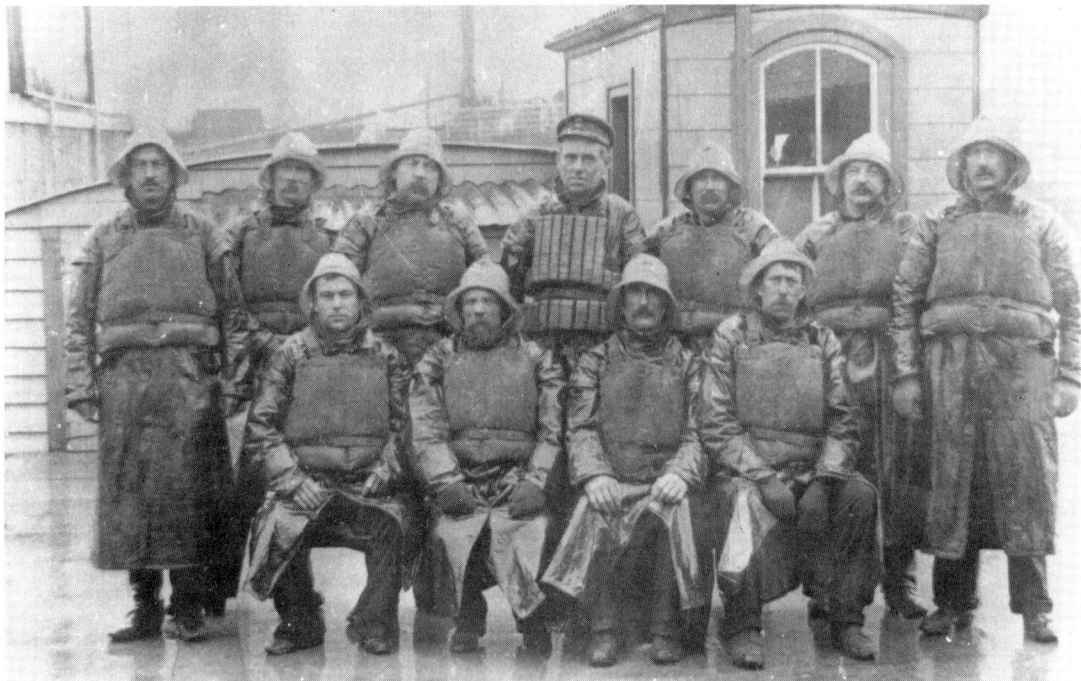

66. This is another fine body of men taken after an excercise. Names leap out of the past: Cuddington, Payne, Holder, Capps, his brother Capps, Cantell, Jones, Clarke, Sandford, Holder... All iron men serving wooden ships!

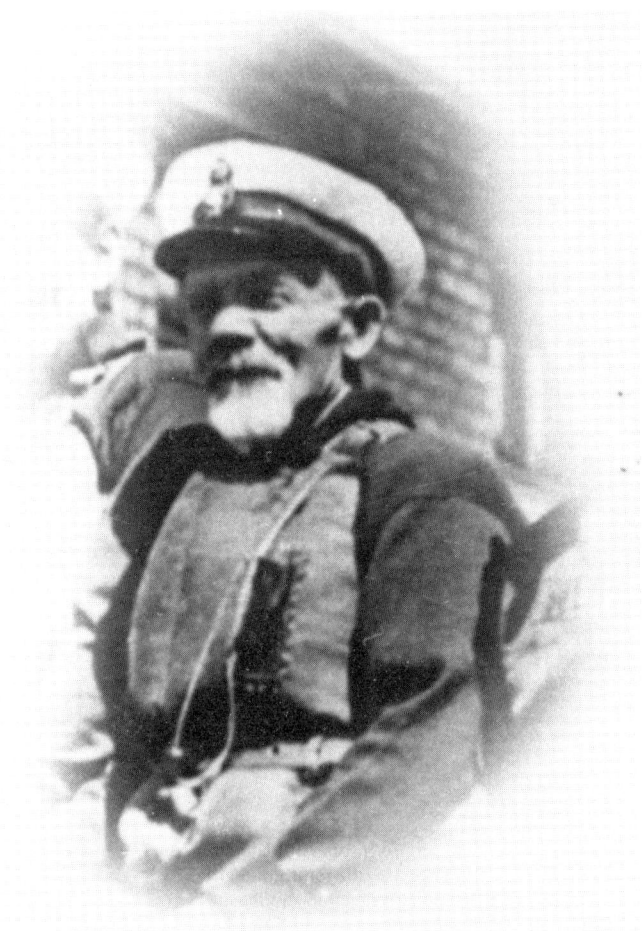

67. Willie 'Rocky' Clarke. On the death of Dick Payne, as we have seen, Rocky Clarke took over as coxswain of the lifeboat. He was the first coxswain of the new lifeboat 'Cecil & Lilian Philpott'. He retired in 1932 having reached the age limit. He had a most remarkable career having twice been shipwrecked. At age 16 he was apprenticed aboard the barque 'Vizcaya'. On arrival at New York he ran away and made voyages in a Nova Scotia vessel, after a varied career during which he again took 'french leave'. He was on board the brig 'Mariner', which was run down off the Royal Sovereign, he landed safely at Newhaven. He was mate for 12 years on the collier 'Amanda' and then captain of the 'Isabella Wilson'. She was run down of South Shields. After that exploit Mr. Clarke settled down at Newhaven.

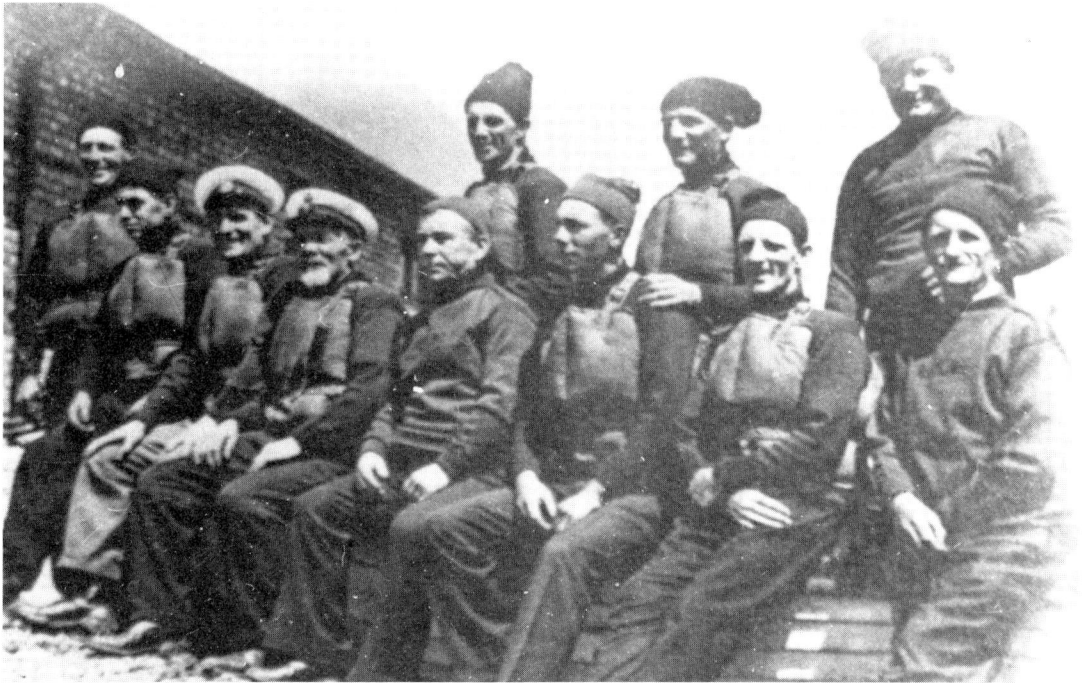

68. Naming ceremony 'Cecil & Lilian Philpott' lifeboat. Jack Ennis, Fred Parker, Dick Lower, Rocky Clarke, Buff Jones, Jack Clarke, George Winder, Sandy Sandford and Cuddington.

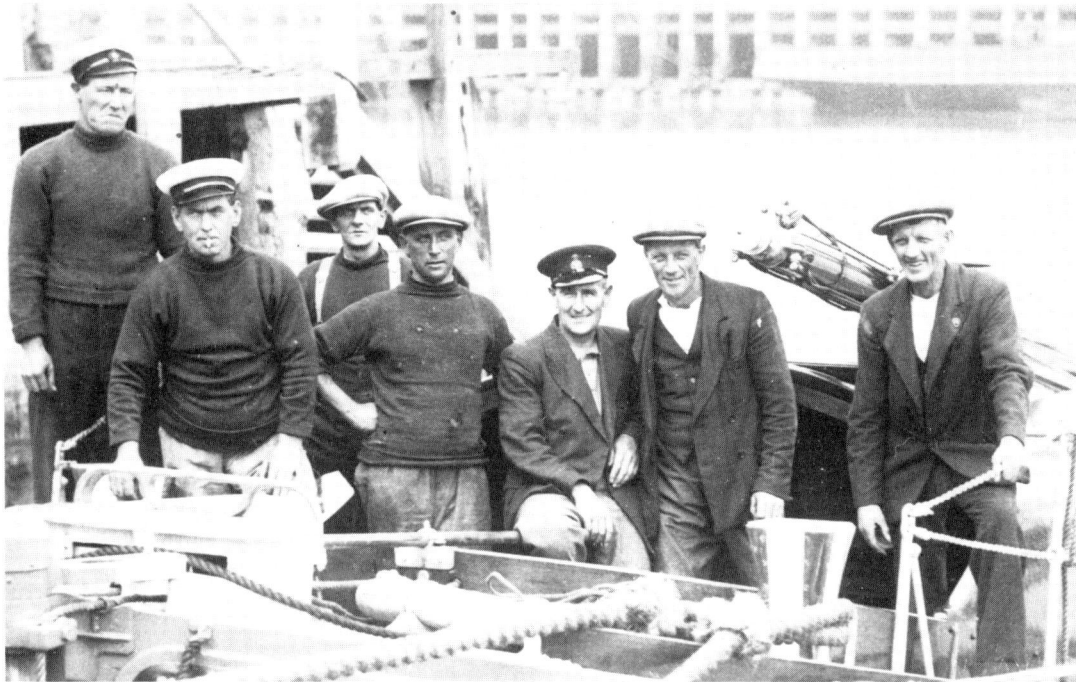

69. 'Cecil & Lilian Philpott' returning from a rescue. Left to right: Tom Hill, a very fine coxswain, Fred Parker, Jack Eager, George Stockwell, Dick Lower, 'Phyllis' Clarke and Jack Clarke... a fine body of men under any circumstances.

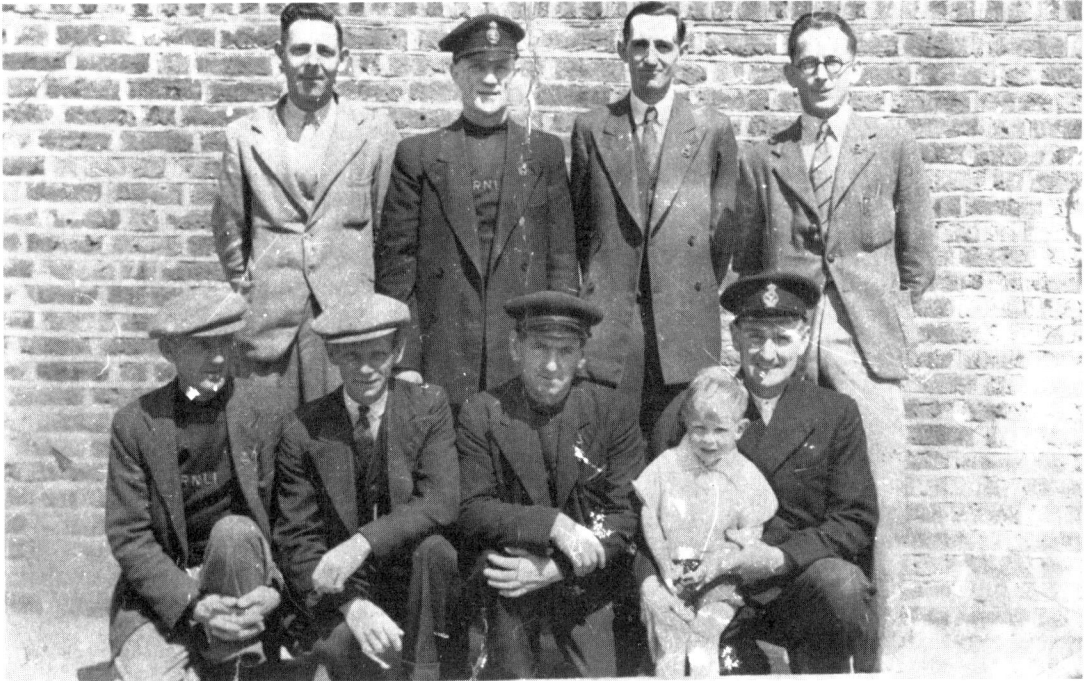

70. Wartime lifeboatmen at Newhaven. This photograph was taken in Gibbon Road, by the wall of the 'Sheffield Arms'. A good many old names come from the past and not so distant past: Bill Sweatman, coxswain 'Phyllis' Clarke, Bob Holden, (head launcher) Dick Sayers, (Hon. Secretary) Dick Lower seen with his son (Bob) Shad Wood and so on.

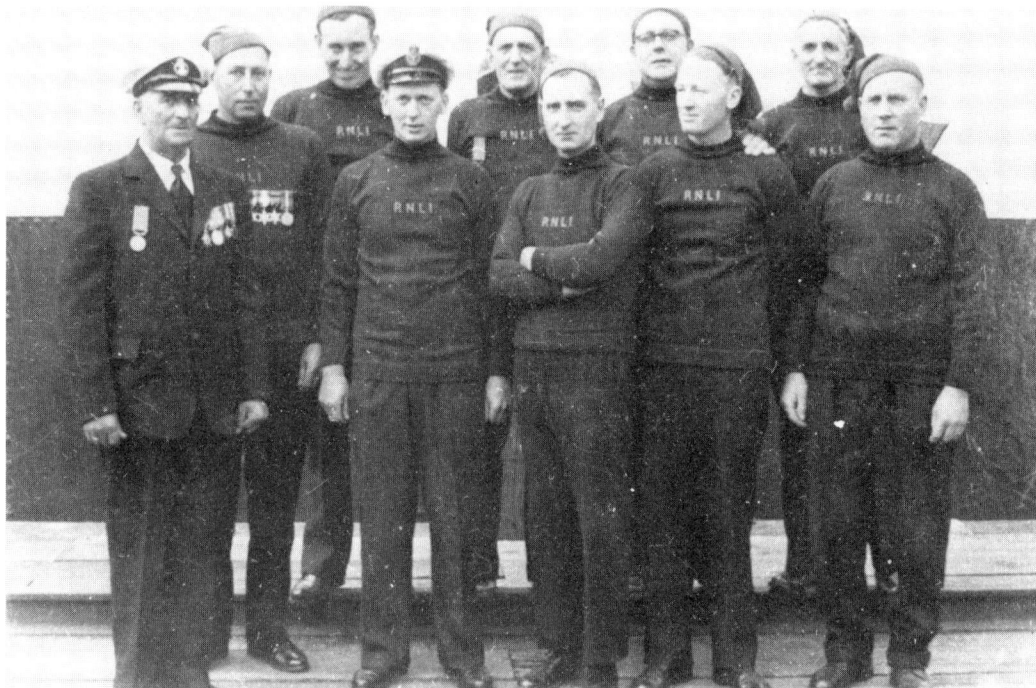

71. Crew photograph 'Cecil & Lilian Philpott'. This was taken after the exploit to the rescue of the crew of the trawler 'Avanturine'. Left to right: coxswain Bill Harvey, Edgar Moore, Harold Moore, Eric Page, 'Nat' Holden, Frank Vacher, 'Trotter' Hills, Bob Derne, Bob Holden, Reg Ingram… a fine turn out…

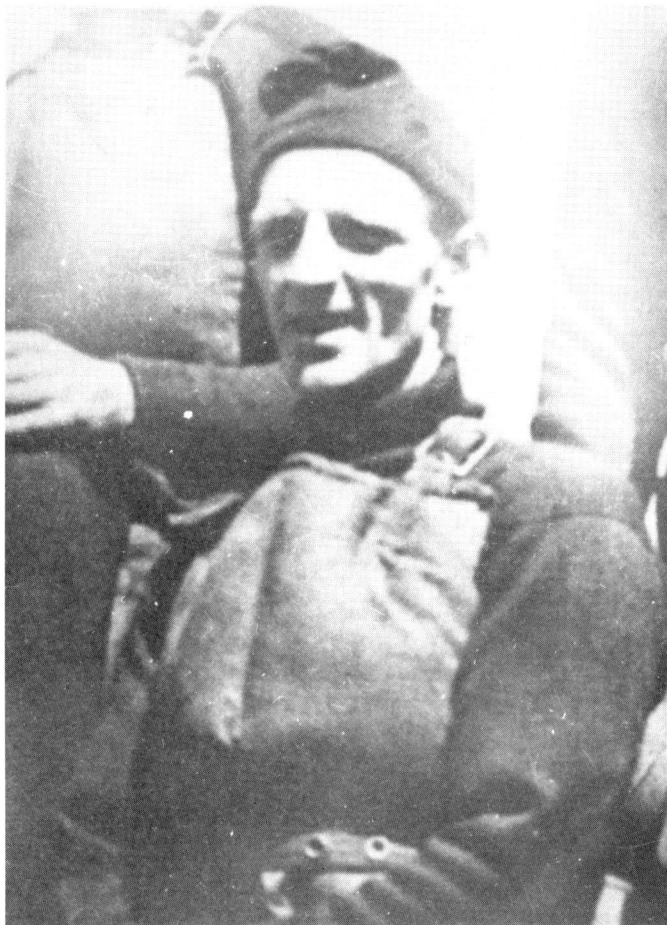

72. Benjamin 'Deafy' Clarke. So called because he was, in fact, all but deaf. He served as signalman on the 'Sir Fitzroy Clayton' lifeboat and later on the 'Cecil & Lilian Philpott'. He was washed overboard and lost in 1943 when the lifeboat went to the assistance of a trawler, 'Avanturine'. The trawler ran into the lifeboat causing considerable damage to the boat and injuring many of the crew. Although a thorough search was made, 'Deafy' could not be found and his body was recovered two days later at Cuckmere.

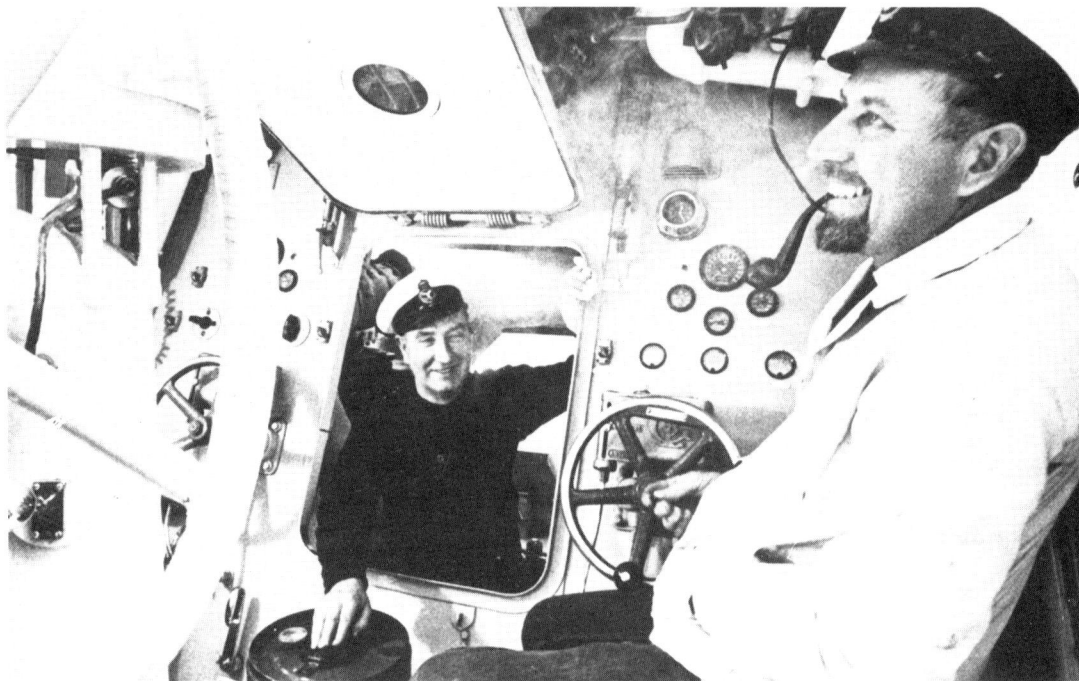

73. Well — there's no point in crying'. Coxswain Edgar Moore with his engineer (and friend) Frank Vacher aboard the lifeboat 'Kathleen Mary'.